MW00782289

HERMETIC
HERBALISM

HERMETIC HERBALISM

The Art of Extracting Spagyric Essences

JEAN MAVÉRIC

Edited and Translated by R. Bailey

Inner Traditions
Rochester, Vermont

Inner Traditions
One Park Street
Rochester, Vermont 05767
www.InnerTraditions.com

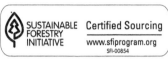

Text stock is SFI certified

English edition and translation copyright © 2020 by R. Bailey

Originally published in French under the title *La médecine hermétique des plantes ou l'extraction des quintessences par art spagyrique* by Dorbon-aîné, Paris, s.d. [1911]

All rights reserved. No part of this book may be reproduced or utilized in any form or by any means, electronic or mechanical, including photocopying, recording, or by any information storage and retrieval system, without permission in writing from the publisher.

Note to the reader: *This book is intended as an informational guide. The remedies, approaches, and techniques described herein are meant to supplement, and not to be a substitute for, professional medical care or treatment. They should not be used to treat a serious ailment without prior consultation with a qualified health-care professional.*

Cataloging-in-Publication Data for this title is available from the Library of Congress

ISBN 978-1-62055-985-7 (print)
ISBN 978-1-62055-986-4 (ebook)

Printed and bound in the United States by Lake Book Manufacturing, Inc. The text stock is SFI certified. The Sustainable Forestry Initiative® program promotes sustainable forest management.

10 9 8 7 6 5 4 3 2 1

Text design and layout by Debbie Glogover
This book was typeset in Garamond Premier Pro with Alchemion, Gill Sans MT Pro, and Segoe UI Symbol used as display fonts

To send correspondence to the translator of this book, mail a first-class letter to the translator c/o Inner Traditions • Bear & Company, One Park Street, Rochester, VT 05767, and we will forward the communication.

For

F.-C. Barlet,

whose knowledge is equaled only by his modesty,

and

my friend Dr. J.-P. Vergnes,

whose noble mission became the realization of this Work.

— J.M.

Contents

PART TWO
ELEMENTARY CHEMISTRY, SPAGYRICS, AND SECRET OPERATIONS

PART THREE
HELMONTIAN MEDICINE AND THE PREPARATION OF ALKAHESTS AND MENSTRUAL VEHICLES

Abbreviations and Symbols, Tables, and Figures

Abbreviations and Symbols

Angles

Asc — Ascendant
MC — Midheaven
Dsc — Descendant
IC — Nadir

Aspects

♂ — Conjunction
☍ — Opposition
□ — Quadrature

Elements

⌔ — Air
△ — Fire
⎹ — Earth
▽ — Water

Luminaries

☉ — Sun
☾ — Moon

Planets

♄ — Saturn
♃ — Jupiter
♂ — Mars

♀ — Venus
☿ — Mercury
♅ — Uranus
♆ — Neptune

Signs of the Zodiac

♈ — Aries
♉ — Taurus
♊ — Gemini
♋ — Cancer
♌ — Leo
♍ — Virgo
♎ — Libra
♏ — Scorpio
♐ — Sagittarius
♑ — Capricorn
♒ — Aquarius
♓ — Pisces

Qualities

H — Hot
W — Wet
C — Cold
D — Dry

Tables

Figures

Translator's Foreword

L ittle is known about the life of Jean Mavéric except that he was a prominent figure in occult and alchemical circles in Paris in the early twentieth century. He was affiliated with Papus's *École hermétique* (formerly the *Groupe indépendant d'études ésotériques*), which offered courses on a wide range of esoteric subjects. Advertisements for the *École hermétique* identify him as a professor of Hermetic philosophy and practical astrology. He was also an active member of the *Société alchimique de France,* a group of occultists devoted to the study and revival of alchemy, founded by François Jollivet-Castelot (1874–1937), to whom Mavéric dedicated his book on ancient alchemy.[1]

Mavéric authored at least ten books between the years 1910 and 1913. According to occult bibliographer Albert Louis Caillet (1869–1928), the name Jean Mavéric is a partial anagram of the author's real name, Maurice Petitjean.[2] What is certain is that "Jean Mavéric" also published under the pseudonyms "Jean Petit" and "Jean Bélus." Jean Petit's *The Key to the Diurnal Horoscope*, originally published circa 1913, was subsequently reprinted under the name Jean Mavéric,[3] and the same is true of the two titles originally published under the pseudonym Jean Bélus in 1911.[4] "Bélus" or *Belus,* by the way, is the Latinate form of the Grecized name Βῆλος, the euhemerized king who established the order of astrologer-priests known as "Chaldeans."[5]*

Belus and Βῆλος are ultimately Latinized and Grecized forms of the name of the Babylonian deity Bel or Baal, meaning "lord," "master," or "possessor."

Mavéric's use of the pseudonym "Jean Petit," a complete and more readily discernable anagram of the author's reputed surname, corroborates Caillet's assertion, but the extensive catalog of esoteric literature compiled by the Parisian bookseller Dorbon-aîné, who published Mavéric's *Hermetic Herbalism* in 1911, makes no mention of the author's first name. Instead, the catalog identifies Jean Mavéric only as "the pseudonym of Petitjean."[6] It is to be noted, however, that the anagrammatic method of devising a pseudonym to which Caillet alludes was especially popular among esotericists in fin-de-siècle France. To cite just one example, Albert Faucheux (1838–1921), the head of the French chapter of the Hermetic Brotherhood of Luxor, created his pseudonym François-Charles Barlet (who is one of the dedicatees of this book) by scrambling the letters of his first name Albert and making this anagram the last name of his pen name F.-C. Barlet. In the exact same manner, Petitjean scrambled the letters of his first name, Maurice, and made this anagram the last name of his preferred nom de plume Jean Mavéric, the letters *U* and *V* being interchangeable not only in Latin but also in early French. This would seem to lend further credence to Caillet's identification. In fact, the only reasonable conclusion one may draw is that Albert Caillet, a Hermeticist in his own right, who wrote the preface to André Durville's French translation of *The Kybalion,* must have known Petitjean personally.[7]

On the basis of Mavéric's scathing critique of the medical field of his day in the preface to *Hermetic Herbalism,* it is also reasonable to assume that he himself was a medical practitioner. His researches into the esoteric sciences may well have been prompted by medical colleagues such as Dr. J.-P. Vergnes (the other dedicatee of this book), a practicing homeopathist and a prolific author who published dozens of articles on occult therapeutics, including the serial "Spagyric Medicine," which he co-authored with Mavéric.[8] There was a Dr. Maurice Petitjean, a former Paris hospital intern (*ancien externe des hôpitaux de Paris*) whose medical thesis "On Inguinal Strangulated Hernia in Infants during the First Two Years of Life" was published in 1899 by Vigot frères,[9] the same Parisian publisher who published Jean Mavéric's treatise on astrological medicine some ten years later.[10] Whether this Dr. Maurice Petitjean and the Maurice Petitjean behind the pseudonym Jean Mavéric are the same person remains unclear. In any case the Maurice Petitjean behind the pseudonym Jean Mavéric must surely have been the instructor Petitjean listed among the associate professors and lecturers of the *École supérieure libre des sciences médicales appliquées,* an outgrowth of Papus's *École hermétique.* According to school advertisements Petitjean co-taught the lecture series "Hermetic Medicine" with Dr. Gérard Encausse (alias Papus), Mr. Paul Schmidt (the pseudonym of Edmond Dace), and Dr. M. Druz, author of *A Practical Treatise of Astral Medicine and Therapeutics,*[11] but whereas the advertisements identify many of the medical school's faculty members, Papus included, by their real names and by professional titles such as *docteur en médecine* and *ancien externe des hôpitaux,* Professor Petitjean is rather bizarrely described as *hommes de lettres,* that is, "men of letters," "scholars," or simply "writers." If the plural *hommes* is not a typographical error, it is likely a clever nod to Petitjean's multiple literary pseudonyms.

At any rate, knowing the enigmatic author's true identity does not make him any less elusive. To the contrary, it succeeds only in making him all the more mysterious. Mavéric may justly be described as the "Fulcanelli of modern herbalism," and *Hermetic Herbalism* is widely regarded as his masterpiece. The influential occultist François Jollivet-Castelot, himself an expert in spagyric medicine, reviewed Mavéric's magnum opus in especially glowing terms:

> This learned work of great importance examines the spagyric treatment of plants point by point. . . . No doubt it will be read with keen interest due to the sore lack of modern studies on the subject. Mavéric is extremely well versed in astrological and alchemical matters. Simply put, no other living author could have written such a superb and authoritative disquisition on the Hermetic art of herbal medicine.[12]

The publication of *Hermetic Herbalism,* as Jollivet-Castelot intimates, was groundbreaking in its day.[13] The only contemporary studies of the kind available in French during the early twentieth century were a few scattered chapters in Papus's heavy tomes and Paul Sédir's *Magical Plants: A Concise Guide to Occult Botany.*[14] But whereas Papus and Sédir were concerned primarily with bridging the widening gap between modern botanical studies and the esoteric sciences, Mavéric was concerned with restoring the ancient and often forgotten Hermetic foundations of the science of herbal medicine.

From Mavéric's point of view, the vast majority of modern-day books about herbal alchemy or spagyric medicine are largely, if not entirely, concerned with basic chemistry. This, of course, is not to say that the herbal preparations provided in such books are worthless or ineffectual, only that they are neither Hermetic nor spagyric. For Mavéric the art of extracting herbal essences is not by default spagyric. He defines spagyrics as a series of chemical operations that proceed by analogy from Hermetic principles and universal laws. One of the major distinguishing factors of spagyric operations is *time,* and this extends not only to the protracted duration of the chemical procedures but also to the timing of the planting and harvesting of the vegetal matter. Mavéric states in no uncertain terms that herbal essences extracted by spagyric operations are infinitely more potent and effective than herbal essences extracted by normal chemical procedures. Thus, to distinguish the spagyric essence from the ordinary or "aspagyric," Mavéric consistently utilizes the term *quintessence,* in accordance with the writings of the old spagyrists and alchemists.

A few words are necessary here on some of the editorial changes made in this translation. French esotericists in the early twentieth century were notoriously negligent when it came to properly citing their sources, and Jean Mavéric is no exception. Mavéric makes use of a great number of sources from the fifteenth through the nineteenth centuries, but he cites virtually none of them. I have made every effort to track down all of his Latin and French sources and to cite them accordingly in the annotations (along with any existing English translations of these sources).

Furthermore, due to the nature and extent of Mavéric's sources, there is little consistency in the original French publication with respect to plant names. Mavéric frequently employs a variety of different French common names and partial scientific names to refer to the same plant genera or species. For example, bear's-breech (*Acanthus mollis* L.) appears as both *blanche-ursine* ("white-ursine") and *acanthe,* from the Latin plant name *acanthus,* which derives from the Greek ἄκανθα ("thorn" or "spine"), dandelion (*Taraxacum officinale* L.) appears as both *dent-de-lion* ("lion's tooth") and *pissenlit* ("piss-the-bed"), the latter being a colorful description of the plant's well-known diuretic properties, and turmeric (*Cucurma longa* L.) appears as both *safran oriental* ("oriental saffron") and *cucurma,* which derives from the Sanskrit *kuṅkumam,* the name of the turmeric-based powder most often applied to the sixth or "third eye" chakra. I have simplified the matter by utilizing one English common name per genus or species.

In addition, since I suspect some readers may require a more precise taxonomy, I have compiled two plant indices for the 618 plants Mavéric mentions. Each index includes the common names used throughout this translation and their modern scientific equivalents. I have structured the plant indices in such a manner that if readers know a particular plant by a different common name than the one used in this translation, they may look up its scientific name online or in a botanical dictionary and then find it in the "Index of Scientific Plant Names," where they will find in parentheses the one equivalent English common name used consistently throughout this book. I have also alphabetized all of the plant lists in chapters 2, 3, 5, and 6 so that readers may use the plant indices with greater facility.

Mavéric describes *Hermetic Herbalism* as a thoroughgoing, expanded, and considerably improved revision of his earlier *Synthetic Essay on Astrological and Spagyric Medicine.* But even so, in a few places he glosses over materials and simply refers readers to this earlier work. Since Mavéric's *Synthetic Essay* remains untranslated, I have filled in these few lacunae for the sake of readers who do not know French. For example, Mavéric's groupings of foods and drinks according to their elemental qualities in chapter 9 now contain all of the ingredients originally listed in his *Synthetic Essay* together with each of the supplements and updates provided in *Hermetic Herbalism.* Lastly, I have arranged Mavéric's original section divisions into chapters and reordered some of the headers, particularly in chapters 9 and 15, for the sake of greater continuity and fluidity.

One final word. Mavéric admits in the afterword that he gives short shrift to some of the physical and practical aspects of spagyrics. For readers who wish to pursue these matters further, Manfred M. Junius's *Spagyrics: The Alchemical Preparation of Medicinal Essences, Tinctures, and Elixirs* (3rd ed., Rochester, Vt: Inner Traditions, 2007) is an excellent place to start.

☉ IN ♉, ☾ IN ♓,

A LARGE AND DENSELY WOODED ISLAND,

R. BAILEY

R. BAILEY received a Doctor of Philosophy degree in Religion in 2017. His research interests include ancient, medieval, and modern traditions of herbalism, magic, Hermeticism, and Gnosticism. He is currently working on translations of Paul Sédir's *Les plantes magiques* and the Latin *Herbarium* of Pseudo-Apuleius.

Author's Preface

Ancient medicine had several loosely connected factions. The Galenic doctrine gathered the greatest number of partisans, but among them there were many injudicious physicians whose "knowledge" consisted in amassing large quantities of absurd *receptes* and *formulae* lacking any scientific foundation. In short, a multitude of ignorant, deceitful, pretentious, and shrewd doctors came to shelter themselves under the umbrella of Galenism. The latter reigned supreme, occupied the highest offices, and published countless works in which they ostentatiously displayed the culpable error of their inane teachings. The unprecedented manner in which such mortal physicians treated King Louis XIII proves that they had access to some of the most powerful figures in history and that their patients were mere dupes.* However, while these potentates of ignorance shone in society, here and there a few modest scientists continued to work diligently in the shadows. Despising success and devoted to science, these humble seekers succeeded in reconstructing the founding principles of the venerable doctrine revealed by Hermes Trismegistus.

Hermetic doctrine encompasses the knowledge of the origins of creation, and therefore of first and second causes and their analogies. It was this doctrine that gave birth to the theory and practice of alchemy and this same doctrine that gave rise to the practices of Hermetic herbalism, iatrochemistry, and medical mineralogy.

---

*By the year of his death in 1643, King Louis XIII had been bled 98 times and had taken 228 purgatives by order of his private doctor.

Only a few rare adepts possessed knowledge of the Hermetic science. Moreover, in order not to defile the secrets of their arduous labors, they wrote very little, and what little they did write was expressed in obscure and veiled language. If one is of the opinion that most people, scholars included, often consider only the surface of things, it should come as no surprise to discover that the works of the spagyrists remain unrecognized today, lost as they were among a cumbersome mass of books published by myopic mountebanks.

The present-day ignorance of Hermetic medicine therefore derives from a combination of two factors: the scarcity and obscurity of the Hermetic writings, and the difficulty the uninitiated have in distinguishing these writings from a multitude of erroneous publications. Given these factors, it would be rash and pretentious for anyone to draw any conclusion regarding this forgotten science *before understanding it.*

Our personal work in this field, conducted in rare book and manuscript libraries and guided by natural inclinations, allows us state emphatically that modern allopathic medicine does not rest on any solid foundation and that it is merely an ephemeral illusion when compared to the Hermetic medicine of the ancients, whose fundamental principles constitute a formidable synthesis that embraces the work of Universal Generation in its entirety.

Spagyric herbal essences combine a powerful virtue with an advanced atomic constitution that is perfectly assimilable to our human nature. On the contrary, the remedies employed in modern allopathy are only raw, undeveloped, and indigestible chemical products whose rudimentary atomic constitution is opposed to the delicate nature of the human body, which can assimilate them only painfully. Moreover, due to their impure constitution, in addition to what little virtue they possess, these chemical products are often not without danger to patients.

Modern allopathy consists of a series of superficial observations based on isolated effects that have no fundamental affinities, lack a comprehensive synthesis, and do not rest on a firm foundation. Such a "medicine" is not a science but merely a heap of provisional, indeterminate, and uncoordinated facts that do not proceed from a clearly defined methodology and, as a result, are destined to dismantle each other. Besides, these painful truths have not escaped the notice of many conscientious and illustrious representatives of this illusory therapeutics, whose opinions are well documented and readily accessible, and hence unnecessary to enumerate here.[1]

Intelligent and conscientious physicians, practitioners, and non-professionals should read this work attentively and without bias. If the astrological components should turn them off, we recommend that they abandon these chapters temporarily and consult the thorough study of the temperaments first. As for the spagyric preparations, which require a great deal of time, care, and patience as well as special installations, many will not be able to put them into practice immediately. In this case, one should in the interim make use of modern homeopathic remedies, which are infinitely superior to their allopathic counterparts. We have written this work in the hope that doctors may someday have a fighting chance to fulfill their oath in good faith.

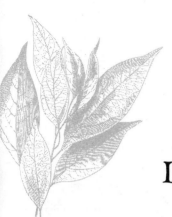

Introduction

The adjective *Hermetic* derives from the modern Latin *hermeticus*, after Hermes Trismegistus, the Egyptian Moses whose colossal science illuminated antiquity with divine light. The term *hermeticus*, however, much like *occultus* (literally, "hidden" or "secret"), actually means "closed" or "invisible," which is to say, it is a science that is closed and invisible to the unclean and to the blind, for only those whose eyes have beheld the Light of Truth may cross the threshold of the Hermetic Sanctuary.

For most authors, the adjective *spagyric*—from the Late Latin *spagyricus*, a portmanteau of the Greek verbs σπᾶν, "to draw," and ἀγείρειν, "to assemble"—means "to purify by resolution." According to Gerardus Johannes Vossius, this Latinate compound means "to concretize rarefied matter,"[1] in other words, to ameliorate the Substance in the evolutive state (or first matter) in order to purify other matter with the aid of the resultant. On the other hand, according to Nicolas de Locques, "spagyric physician" to King Louis XIV, the term *spagyrie* signifies "quicksilver" and refers to the art of separating Mercury from bodies.[2] Be that as it may, we understand the term to refer to any chemical operation that proceeds by analogy from natural laws. To separate Mercury is to extract spirit from matter, to extract the quintessential from the corporeal. All bodies are composed of matter and spirit. Matter is passive and inert, whereas spirit is an active and vital principle imbued with the Divine Thought, the prime mover in the evolutionary process. It is clear, then, that the virtue of mixed bodies resides in the

1

spirit and that the spirit is much more active when it is freed from its corporeal prison.

The entire physical side of the spagyric art is concerned with this separation or extraction. To obtain the spirit at its maximum virtue, it must be exalted, and in order to exalt it, it is necessary to mature (or *evolve*) and ripen it, in other words, to corrupt its body, the way a seed must putrefy in the ground before it is able to germinate. This putrefaction is nothing other than the *evolution of matter,* by which the atoms of a given substance separate themselves from heterogeneities; constrict, purify, and exalt themselves; and elevate themselves to a much more noble latitude than that of their primitive state. The whole of the spagyric art consists in provoking the evolution of matter in order to purify and exalt it, and this is achievable solely through the subtle and protracted operations the old spagyrists left hidden in the shadows of obscurity.

Spagyric preparations accord with the natural mechanisms of Universal Generation. An understanding of these mechanisms will enable the practitioner to extract powerful quintessences whose atomic constitution is so ennobled as to be readily assimilable to our human nature. Such quintessences penetrate the human organism and purify it in a natural and harmonic manner. The ancient sages understood the nature of first and second causes, from which they deduced via synthesis their effects and analogies in the lower world. In this manner they came to understand the process of the alchemical work, which is the analogical reproduction of Universal Generation in the mineral kingdom, a subject concerning which even the most accomplished modern scholars have understood next to nothing.

Hermetic herbalism is based on the knowledge of universal laws, first in their intimate nature and then in their effects and analogies. It is essential that the practitioner know the nature of the astral and elemental influences as well as what causes are likely to modify the nature of these influences. In addition, the practitioner cannot ignore the effects these influences have on the organized world or the analogical correspondences that unite the macrocosm with the microcosm.

All this knowledge constitutes a synthesis that is at once simple, grandiose, and subtle. It is *simple* because its laws are the laws of nature, by which human beings were created. It is *grandiose* because it embraces the evolutionary process of the whole of creation. It is *subtle* because its intimate conception cannot be grasped by human reason, which is limited to our imperfect control of the physical senses and obscured by the errors inherent in social education. To acquire any notion, one must understand not only its purpose, function, and form (which is the domain of reason), but also, and above all, one must ingest and digest its intimate spirit, by way of the soul, until it is completely assimilated. In short, one must penetrate the nature of the thing, *to the point of living it within oneself.*

The practice of this secret path requires that the student show a natural inclination to grow and develop gradually, by a long process of evolution, or rather, involution, on an ascending course that leads from *impure* to *pure*, from *dross* to *divine*. In other words, it is necessary to free the soul from its carnal prison by delivering it from the demands of egoism, by breaking the ties that bind it to the instinct, and by purifying oneself constantly on the physical, psychical, and intellectual planes.

Physical purification can be achieved through the daily use of foods of an exclusively vegetal origin and through chaste morals. *Psychical* purification can be developed through the practice of disinterestedness, which consists in performing works of charity and humility and in keeping for oneself only what is necessary to live a normal, simple, and modest lifestyle. Persistent contemplation of the works of NATURE combined with an enlightened religious outlook will confer on the disciple notions of the TRUE, the GOOD, and the BEAUTIFUL. *Intellectual* purification can be obtained through the progressive, patient, and persistent practice of a well-balanced Will that aims to purge the self of the judgments, perceptions, errors, conceptions, habits, prejudices, and conventions inherent in social life and in the outside world. In this manner practitioners may gradually elevate the framework of their conceptions to first and second causes. This tripartite sublimation is absolutely necessary to release the rays of the Intellective Light by which initiates gain entry into the Hermetic Sanctuary.

The science of Hermetic herbalism is much less arid than that of

Hermetic mineralogy, which includes the alchemical work. So-called erudition, which overloads the memory with a host of details and conventions, is useless in this art. Curiosity, on the other hand, can be extremely hazardous if it is not legitimated by a pure and disinterested conscience. In sum, to attain this great knowledge one must free oneself from preconceived notions and contingencies and study patiently, modestly, and humbly, starting with the rigorous examination of oneself.

To conclude this brief introduction, we would like to stress to our readers that this book is no mere compilation, despite the numerous authors we consulted in the process of writing it. The works of the masters are comparable to *matter,* from which readers must extract the *quintessence.**

---

*The present work represents not only a substantial revision of our earlier work, *Essai synthétique,* but also a considerable improvement of it. The process of Universal Generation is here more clearly developed and complete, and the same is true of the correspondences of plants to the planets and the signs of the zodiac. The system of astral vibrations and their effects and analogies is here definitively resolved, and it should therefore replace the system outlined in *Essai synthétique,* which was only intended to be provisional. Furthermore, spagyric operations are here clearly exposed, whereas those described in *Essai synthétique* remain incomplete. Notwithstanding, our *Essai synthétique* still contains valuable information concerning the study of the temperaments, the investigation of diseases, and the elemental analysis of plants.

PART ONE

Universal Generation, Plants, Hermetic Medicine, and Astral Influences

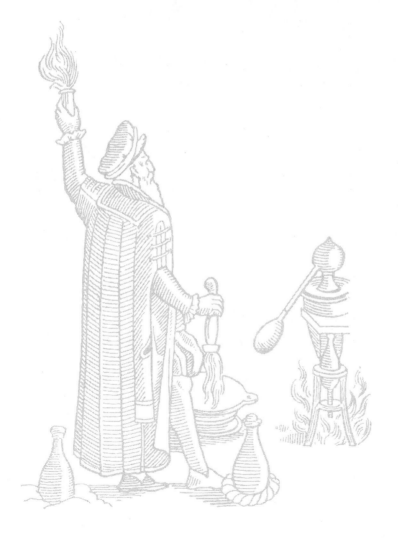

1
Synthesis of the Origins of Creation

The *One Ethereal Substance* is an imprint of the Divine Thought, the eternal origin of the harmonized force. It fills space with its cold and white radiation from innumerable sources that speckle the infinite. *Essential Light* issues forth from these multiple centers of *First Thought* in negative vibrations that extend in all directions, intersecting and colliding in inharmonic modes of a positive nature. These dissonances produce vortices whose speed of rotation increases until the production of red heat becomes Fire. In this manner energy centers are formed which contain the embryonic principle of the laws of creation.

As soon as they are formed, these igneous whirlwinds are drawn by indeterminate attractions and travel an indefinite spiraliform path until reaching a point of equilibrium. But the immutable law of inertia, whose principle is the centripetal force, opposes isolated motion, and thus the heat of these potential centers gradually diminishes together with their speed of rotation. It is at this stage that energy pours forth from the *One Substance* and condenses until it transforms into a formless matter.

To set its evolution in motion, this chaotic matter gradually acquires a certain negative vibration of a quaternary nature. This vibration manifests in four distinct modes, which are the four elemental qualities: hot, wet, cold, and dry. These qualities therefore constitute the state of transition by which the *Original Substance* coalesces into positive principles, for the elements of creation are born of the coupling of these qualities, and evolutionary life sits at the center of the four elements that emitted from the primal chaos.

The Formation of the Four Elements

To fully understand how the elements formed, it is necessary first to discuss their qualitative combinations and to examine their particular natures.

Hotness is neither wet nor dry, but simply hot in nature, fluidic, expansive, dynamic, dilative, and positive: it is the origin of the *masculine principle.* Wetness is neither hot nor cold, but naturally volatile, subtle, attenuating, moderating, vaporous, and fleeting: it is the origin of the *feminine principle.* Coldness is neither wet nor dry, but naturally cold, fixative, inert, conservative, and concentrative: it is the origin of the *principle of fixation and atony.* Dryness is neither hot nor cold, but naturally desiccating, sterile, arid, reactive, erethitic, and irritative: it is the origin of the *principle of retention and opposition.*

The element Fire (△) is born of exaltation, from the action of the *dry* on the *hot,* which concentrates it and makes it violent and active. Fire in isolation is naturally violent, active, destructive, combustive, and diffusive. The element Air (⩟) is born of the action of the *hot* on the *wet,* which exalts, dilates, and volatilizes it. Isolated Air has a harmonic, generative, temperate, and maturing nature. The element Water (∇) is born of the action of the *cold* on the *wet,* which condenses, retains, and weighs it down. Water in isolation is naturally passive, attenuating, unstable, disintegrative, dispersive, and receptive. The element Earth (⩝) is born of the action of the *dry* on the *cold,* which divides it and opposes its coagulation due to its reactive nature. Isolated Earth is naturally neutral, inert, concentrative, arid, and absorptive.

Universal Generation

Fire is the dynamic principle of the generative process, which it furnishes with spontaneous impulse. It generates motion and action and is imbued with igneous soul. *Air* tempers the violence of Fire, harmonizes motion, and measures action. It fertilizes Earth and Water, giving rise to putrefaction, a process which always precedes generation. *Water* volatilized by Fire falls as rain upon Earth to circulate and corrupt upon it germs fertilized by Air and animated by Fire. Water causes putrefaction on Earth through the intermediation of Air. *Earth* receives the animation of Fire by means of the dry and the fertilization of Air through the agency of Water, which causes putrefaction upon it, as in a matrix. Earth is the receptor for fertilized germs.

The process of generation therefore takes place in Earth and in Water, putrefied by Air and animated by Fire. Such is the origin of the constituent principles. They alone directly engender the substances of mixed bodies, which are neighbors to matter.

The Origin of the Three Constituent Principles

When Fire (hot and dry) and Air (hot and wet) collide, the dryness of the one and the wetness of the other weaken and become passive, while the common quality of hotness, becoming active, is realized in the material principle of *Sulfur*. When Air (hot and wet) and Water (cold and wet) meet, the hot and the cold attenuate and the shared quality of wetness manifests on the material plane in the form of *Mercury*. When Fire (hot and dry) comes into contact with Earth (cold and dry), the hot and the cold are neutralized, activating the quality of dryness, which generates *Salt*. Finally, when Water (cold and wet) merges with Earth (cold and dry), the wet and the dry qualities are moderated, causing the cold to become the sphere of action. However, since the cold is atonic and anti-vital in nature, it does not generate a constituent principle, and this is why the elements Water and Earth come to be materialized in mixed bodies.

In sum, Sulfur is the materialization of the quality of hotness in Fire and Air, Mercury the materialization of the quality of wetness in Air and Water, and Salt the materialization of the quality of dryness in Fire and Earth. The quality of coldness is unproductive and inhabits the passive elements Water and Earth.

The Distinctive Natures
of the Constituent Principles

Mercury or Spirit is a subtle wetness, volatile, mobile, spiritual, essential, and generative in nature. It is the feminine principle of the seed, passive in generation in relation to Sulfur, but active in its mobility. Mercury resides in Water, its vehicle. In the vegetable kingdom it constitutes the spiritual part of the plant and administers its aroma. In the mineral kingdom it is strongly united to Sulfur by Salt.

Sulfur or Soul is a fixed, latent hotness that does not burn but warms gently. It is the dynamic agent of fermentation and the male principle of the seed, active in generation in relation to Mercury. Sulfur is naturally hot, digestive, stimulating, and fertilizing. Its intrinsic hotness causes the evolution of matter and fights against the atonic action of the cold. It resides in Salt, which more or less retains and thickens it. In the vegetable kingdom it manifests in the forms of the essence, oil, resin, and sap of the plant. It resides in the warm, essential, and heady parts of plants and generates their flavor.

Salt or Body is a negative principle that is desiccative, condensing, reactive, and coagulative in nature. It thickens the mercurial water, which dissolves it, and fixes Sulfur in Earth. Salt intimately unites Sulfur with Mercury. It is the principle of conservation and opposes corruption.

These three constituent principles are found in vulgar Water and Earth, which serve as their matrices, vehicles, and bases. The processes of fermentation and fertilization occur naturally in Water and Earth.

The World Spirit

The *Divine-Uncreated-Eternal Thought* is the origin of all creation, and all vibrations emanating from the First Thought are virtual imprints of it. The Divine Spirit accompanies the work of creation in the evolutive process the Substance undergoes and becomes realized in matter by identifying itself with the individual nature of the various states through which it passes over the course of its evolution.

The Divine Thought manifests in the process of Universal Generation in the form of a *vital-active spirit* nascent in a *hot-aerial wetness,* which is *the origin of all generation,* for life is born in the center of double polarities whose principle resides in the hot and wet qualities (female and male, Mercury and Sulfur). This active spirit, the principle of vitality and ideal form, resides in Mercury and Sulfur, which Salt unites with matter. When the spagyrist extracts it from mixed bodies, it is imprinted with the nature of the three constituent principles *in a single form* called "quintessence."

The quintessence is therefore an active spiritual substance made up of spirit and soul, united by volatile Salt, and animated by the *Spiritus Mundi* or World Spirit. The spagyric art seeks to extract this substance from matter in order to regenerate the human body or ennoble imperfect metals.

The Process of Universal Generation According to the Numerical Laws of the Kabbalah

1. The *Unity* represents the synthesis of the Divine Thought and the origin of the universe. It is the Divine-Uncreated-Eternal Thought, which individualizes matter by form.

2. The *Binary* is the negative First Thought realized in a positive mode. It represents the union of soul and body, active and passive, male and female, Sulfur and Mercury, matter animated by spirit, the fixed and the volatile.

3. The *Ternary* represents the number of creation, the image of the Divine Trinity, the three states of matter (spirit, soul, and body), the three generative qualities (wet, hot, and dry), and the three constituent principles (Mercury, Sulfur, and Salt).

4. The *Quaternary* represents the number of universal equilibrium, the Unity manifested in the Ternary, the four creative elements, the four seasons of the year, and the four phases of the Moon.

5. The *Quinary* denotes the First Thought in the quintessence, which animates the four elements.

6. The *Senary* signifies the realization of the spiritual Ternary in the physical Ternary, the three generative qualities in the three constituent principles, and the union of the Binary with the Quaternary.

7. The *Septenary* symbolizes the synthetic number of the universe: the

seven astral natures, the Senary animated by the Universal Spirit, the Ternary manifested in the Quaternary, and the union of the Binary and the Quinary.

Perfect knowledge of the relational laws of these numbers in the work of creation will open the door of the Hermetic Sanctuary to the student.

The Anatomical Constitution of the Universal Elements

The elemental and astral influences are of dual and diverse natures. Some are negative and latent, while others are positive and actual. Each active or passive sphere of influence has, in addition to its elemental nature, an intimate nature of its own.

The effects of these potentialities are pure and natural only at certain times and only in certain positions or places, namely those which provide the most appropriate conditions for the manifestation of their influence. The modification or transition from one nature to another generates an element of an intermediary nature, which participates in the one and the other and unites them. In nature, every transition, modification, and transformation occurs smoothly and harmonically.

This proves that the *traditional* succession of the elemental natures of the zodiacal signs is misguided, because there is no transition in this schema between the Fire signs and the Water signs, nor between the Air signs and the Earth signs, whose natures are diametrically opposed. The dual nature of the signs is pure only at their midpoint (15th degree) and weakens at their extremities in order to unite with their conjunct sign *without any solution of continuity*. The elemental natures of the four positions of the Sun in a twenty-four-hour period and over the course of the year succeed each other in the order of nature, and this shows that the true order of the succession of the signs should be as follows: Air → Fire → Earth → Water. The four aspects of the Moon to the Sun are subject to the same natural law, as we shall demonstrate later.

Each season is pure *only at its midpoint*. The *equinoctial* and *solsticial* points represent the center of the transitional natures that unite the four seasons or four elements via the four qualities hot, wet, cold, and dry.* Detailed correspondences for each of the four elements are provided in Table 1.1 (on page 16).

Ettmüller's Classification of Plants

The following classification belongs to the German physician Michael Ettmüller (1644–1683), who was a truly gifted chemist. His taxonomy is very general, however, and appears to be based exclusively on essential differences in plant natures, their substance and constitution in particular.

1st Class: aqueous and insipid plants such as purslane, houseleek, lettuce, romaine, and endive, which contain a temperate and hidden alkali salt and are very refreshing. Their essences, due to the alkali salt they contain, precipitate solutions of Saturn made with vinegar.†

2nd Class: aqueous and acidic plants such as sorrel, wood sorrel, and all plants with an acidic flavor. The acidic principle of these plants is retained in a hidden alkali. Their juice is useful for moderating outbreaks of hot bile.

3rd Class: inodorous and bitter-tasting plants containing a subtle nitrous salt such as chicory, blessed thistle, milk thistle, common hop, fumitory, common centaury, and dandelion. The salt extracted from the juice of these plants becomes flammable when sufficiently depurated by washing. These plants are detersive, diuretic, sudorific, eliminative, and depurative.

4th Class: plants with an acrid and penetrating taste such as watercress, scurvy grass, mustard, horseradish, arugula, and pepper. These plants have antiscorbutic properties and correct the acidity of the melancholic temperament.

---

*Some authors attribute to the quality of wetness the nature of Water and to Sulfur that of Fire; others claim that Salt is a frozen Water, because Salt dissolves in Water by deliquium. But this is all nonsense: wetness is a subtle vapor, which becomes Water only when it unites with the cold, which condenses it, but wetness can also become Air when it unites with the hot, which volatilizes it. Sulfur neither burns nor dries like Fire. It is a coagulated hotness that can be both wet and dry. The fact that Salt attracts Water from Air is indisputable proof of its natural dryness.

†[Mavéric refers here to a solution of vinegar impregnated with acetate of lead, a salt composed of acetous acid and white oxide of lead. Acetate of lead was formerly called "sugar of lead," "sugar of Saturn," "salt of Saturn," "vinegar of Saturn," and "extract of Saturn." —*Trans.*]

5th Class: aromatic plants such as sage, rosemary, pennyroyal, wormwood, thyme, wild thyme, lovage, angelica, anise, fennel, and cumin. These plants contain an oily volatile salt that can be extracted by distillation, which is more active than the spirit obtained by fermentation. These plants have a vulnerary, cephalic, stomachic, nervine, uterine, and cordial virtue.[1]

Ettmüller's Classification of Flowers

1st Class: inodorous flowers like water lily, snapdragon, columbine, and cornflower. Their thick juices possess calmative properties.

2nd Class: flowers with a subtle scent such as lily of the valley, rose, violet, and jasmine. Little or no fragrant oil can be extracted from these flowers except by infusion, but such oils are more cosmetic than medicinal.

3rd Class: aromatic flowers such as lavender, thyme, and wild thyme, which possess the same virtues as the plants that bear them.

As for woods, Ettmüller does not make any distinctions between them, for he claims that by the same operations the practitioner can draw out a water, an acid spirit, a coarse, malodorous, and empyreumatic oil, or a fixed salt found in the residue. To be sure, these divisions are somewhat rudimentary, but they are nevertheless not without merit.[2]

Ettmüller's Classification of Seeds

1st Class: seeds with a strong flavor or aroma that are carminative in nature such as fennel, anise, caraway, and cumin, which are commonly prescribed for convulsions and hysteria.

2nd Class: seeds with a strong and acrid taste such as mustard, pepper, and scurvy grass, from which an anti-putrefactive spirit can be extracted by fermentation.

3rd Class: temperate seeds, especially those which may contain an aqueous mucilage, such as parsley, fenugreek, the four greater cold seeds (squash, pumpkin, melon, and cucumber), and the four lesser cold seeds (lettuce, purslane, endive, and chicory). The juice of these seeds is sometimes oily like that of flax seed or sweet almonds.[3]

Le Fèvre's Classification of Seeds

The reader will notice that the classifications of Michael Ettmüller and those of the French chemist and alchemist Nicaise Le Fèvre (1615–1669), although equally useful, differ from each other significantly.

1st Class: mucilaginous and unctuous seeds whose fixed constituent principles yield their virtue more easily by decoction than by distillation.

2nd Class: milky seeds of a whitish and tender substance from which oils may be rendered after they have been properly dried, but whose virtue resides in the emulsion or lacteous substance extracted by expression.

3rd Class: oleaginous and sulfurous seeds that contain little water and are composed of a compact, arid, and astringent substance due to the predominance of a sulfur over the salt. These seeds are suited to yield their virtue by distillation.[4]

Le Fèvre's Classification of Plants

Perennials, Le Fèvre explains, are fortified by the Universal Spirit at the vernal and autumnal equinoxes and in this manner are able to draw nourishment and preserve themselves, whereas annuals, which are not preserved by their roots, must be renewed each year by their seed.[5] These two types of plants are divisible into three classes:

1st Class: inodorous plants, some of which are insipid, acidic, or bitter, while others have a complex flavor and still others have a dominant taste of a sharp and subtle nature. These plants are green and tender, and their virtue begins to appear in the prime of their vegetation because they abound in juices containing an essential tartarous salt, which with time and heat becomes mucilaginous. This juice is difficult to extract if these plants are harvested too late, so they must be gathered *in their succulence,* when they are tender and green and their stem bends and breaks with the slightest effort.

2nd Class: plants whose virtue comes late in their growth. At first, when they are green and tender, they have no flavor or odor and are filled with an elemental water that has the smell of fresh grass. This water contains, in an embryonic state, a spirituous salt and a subtle sulfur whose virtue manifests only when the matured plant is devoid of phlegm, that is, when the flavor and odor of the plant are conspicuous. These plants must be picked when their stem starts to grow dry at the base and their seed begins to appear.

3rd Class: plants whose flavor is evident from the first days of their vegetation, but whose odor is imperceptible except for when their juice has been expressed. Their juice is thick and viscous and contains a bitter and biting salt, but sometimes it can be honeyed and sacchariferous. Their virtue can be extracted only by digestion or by fermentation. These plants should be picked when they are still in bloom *if they are inodorous and bitter;* but if they bear fruits, berries, or grains, it is then necessary to await their maturity, for their principle virtue resides entirely in these fruits.[6]

Le Fèvre's classification of plants is particularly valuable and will be a great asset to practitioners who are adept enough to distinguish which plants belong to each of his three classes, a subject which Le Fèvre regrettably avoids. Such generic typologies are, in any case, insufficient for the treatment of illnesses, which is why the ancient physicians constructed a detailed taxonomy of simples according to the effects they have on the human body and the afflictions they can alleviate or cure. This system of classification differs somewhat from author to author, but it is more or less homogeneous and its principles are firmly established.

TABLE 1.1.
ELEMENTAL CORRESPONDENCES

Subject	Water	Air	Fire	Earth
State	Liquid	Volatile	Fluidic	Solid
Nature	Fluctuation	Harmony	Destruction	Aridity
Function	Circulation	Nutrition	Dynamism	Reception
Action	Attentuation	Moderation	Violence	Reaction
Motion	Reflexive	Normative	Excessive	Retentive
Effect	Disaggregation	Attraction	Diffusion	Concentration
Creation	Putrefaction	Maturation	Animation	Germination
Generation	Female Seed	Male Seed	Fertilization	Gestations
Season	Winter	Spring	Summer	Autumn
Sun	Midnight	Rising	Midday	Setting
Moon	Opposition	First Quarter	Conjunction	Last Quarter
Sentiment	Passivity	Love	Passion	Egoism
Faculties	Inconsistent	Balanced	Brilliant	Profound
Character	Versatility	Judgment	Enthusiasm	Reservation
Age	Childhood	Adulthood	Middle Age	Old Age
Humor	Phlegm	Blood	Yellow Bile	Black Bile
Temperament	Phlegmatic	Sanguine	Choleric	Melancholic
Organ	Stomach	Chest	Head	Legs
Digestion	Neutral	Salty	Alkaline	Acidic
Savor	Insipid	Sweet	Bitter	Sour
Odor	Inodorous	Savory	Robust	Acrid

2
Medicinal Classifications of Simples

First Division in Seven Classes

Class 1.1. Purgatives, Emetics, and Evacuants

Effects: evacuates excremental humors through the natural channels (eliminative in action).

Plants: agaric, aloe, bastard saffron, bistort, black alder, blackthorn, buckthorn, cassia, colocynth, creeping gratiola, cyclamen, dwarf elder, elderberry, flax-leaved daphne, gamboge, ipecacuanha, iris, manna, myrobalan, peach tree, rhubarb, scammony, sea bindweed, senna, simarouba, spurge laurel, sun spurge, tamarind, turpeth, white hellebore, wild cucumber, wild flax, wild teasel.

Class 1.2. Bechics and Pectorals

Effects: calms coughs and evacuates viscous slime in the bronchi.

Plants: almond, benzoin, borage, catsfoot, coltsfoot, common bugloss, cotton plant, date, elecampane, field cotton rose, fig, golden reinette apple, grape, ground ivy, hedge mustard, jujube, licorice, lungwort, maidenhair spleenwort, pineapple, pistachio, red cabbage, rustyback, sulphurwort, sundew, turnip, viper's bugloss.

Class 1.3. Errhines, Sternutatories, and Salivants

Effects: excites the nasal mucosa and sneezing, alleviates migraines, and decongests the head.

Plants: ginger, Indian horse chestnut, licebane, mastic, mustard, oleander, pepper, pyrethrum, rose campion, sneezewort, spurge, tobacco.

Class 1.4. Antihysterics and Emmenagogues

Effects: provokes menstruation (acting in an antibilious, comforting, and nervine manner).

Plants: ammoniacum, asafetida, birthwort, camphor, catnip, chaste tree, galbanum, German chamomile, horehound, Jerusalem oak goosefoot, lemon balm, marigold, mint, mugwort, myrrh, nutsedge, opopanax, rue, saffron, sagapenum, savin, spoon-leaved sundew, stinking goosefoot, sweet flag, valerian, wallflower.

Class 1.5. Aperients and Diuretics

Effects: excites the appetite, provokes urination, and decongests the kidneys, liver, and mesentery.

Plants: Alexanders, artichoke, ash, birch, blue eryngo, broom, burdock, butcher's broom, caper, celery, chickpea, columbine, common cocklebur, common corn cockle, common restharrow, common water crowfoot, couch grass, dandelion, dock, dropwort, fennel, fir, horseradish, Job's tears, juniper, leek, madder, onion, parsley, pasqueflower, purple star thistle, sea fennel, skirret, smooth rupturewort, sorrel, stinking ground pine, strawberry, tamarind, tea plant, turpentine tree, wild celery, wild chicory.

Class 1.6. Diaphoretics and Sudorifics

Effects: eliminates watery and impure principles through the pores of the skin.

Plants: angelica, benzoin, black salsify, boxwood, butterbur, cinnamon, great golden maidenhair, guaiac wood, Indian bulrush, juniper, meadowsweet, milk thistle, olibanum, scabious, sarsaparilla, walnut, water germander, zedoary.

Class 1.7. Cordials and Alexitaries

Effects: comforts the heart, regulates the heartbeat, and prevents syncope and fainting.*

---

*[The old pharmaceutical term "alexitary" has no exact modern equivalent. An alexitary is a form of *preventive* medicine, but more specifically it is an herbal medicine that

Plants: anemone, cardamom, carline thistle, carnation, cashew nut, citron, clove, cubeb pepper, fraxinella, galega, garlic, kermes grains, lemon, leopard's-bane, motherwort, orange, sandalwood, satyrion, spikenard, squill, tarragon, white swallowwort, wood sorrel, xylobalsam, yellow monkshood.

Second Division in Seven Classes

The following plants act passively on the human body. Their effects are less perceptible than the preceding, but their virtues are nonetheless just as effective.

Class 2.1. Alteratives, Cephalics, and Aromatics of the First Order

Effects: restores general functions, equilibrium, and circulation, and balances the humors.

Plants: aloeswood, basil, bay laurel, bedstraw, betony, calamint, cat thyme, chickweed, cinnamon, clove, common mistletoe, foxglove, golden germander, greater galangal, hyssop, lavender, lily of the valley, linden, marjoram, nutmeg, oregano, pennyroyal, peony, primrose, rosemary, sage, savory, storax, thyme, wild cherry, wild thyme.

Class 2.2. Ophthalmics

Effects: suppresses inflammation of the eyes by application, washing, or absorption (acting in a detersive and refreshing manner).

Plants: clover, cornflower, eyebright, forking larkspur, Good King Henry, greater celandine, sarcocolla, vervain, wild teasel.

Class 2.3. Stomachics and Vermifuges

Effects: excites the digestive functions and destroys gastrointestinal parasites.

(*cont. from p. 18*) wards off contagions and infectious diseases. The term derives from the Greek adjective ἀλεξητήριος, meaning "able to keep off, defend, or help." As a neuter substantive, ἀλεξητήριον takes on the meaning of "remedy, medicine, or protection," or even "charm against (a specific disease)." The nearest modern equivalents to alexitaries would be antiviral, antibacterial, or antimicrobial medicines. Cf. Mavéric's comments on the spirit and oil of angelica root in chapter 13. —*Trans.*]

Plants: catechu, coffee, Greek yarrow, mint, santolina, southernwood, tansy, tarragon, vanilla, wormwood.

Class 2.4. Febrifuges
Effects: lowers body temperature and the pulse.
Plants: avens, common centaury, gentian, germander, shepherd's purse, silver cinquefoil, quinine.

Class 2.5. Hepatics and Splenics
Effects: disgorges the liver and spleen of bilious contents and hot humors.
Plants: agrimony, chervil, common hop, cuckoopint, dodder, fern, fiber hemp, fumitory, greater centaury, hart's tongue fern, hemp agrimony, liverwort, polypody, tarragon.

Class 2.6. Carminatives
Effects: breaks up and dissolves viscous and thick substances and raw humors.
Plants: anise, bishop's weed, caraway, chamomile, coriander, dill, hartwort, lovage, parsnip, star anise, stone parsley, wild carrot, yellow sweet clover.

Class 2.7. Antiscorbutics
Effects: lenifies, tonifies, and asepticizes the tissues, lubricates the mucous membranes, and divides thick humors in the blood.
Plants: arugula, brooklime, creeping jenny, horseradish, nasturtium, pepper cress, scurvy grass, shellac, turmeric, water clover, watercress, water dock, water parsnip, white cinnamon.

Third Division in Seven Classes
Class 3.1. Alteratives of the Second Order
Effects: purifies and tightens the tissues and divides congealed and fixed humors (anti-traumatic in action).
Plants: acacia, amaranth, balsam of Peru, barberry, bistort, bloody dock, bugle, cinquefoil, common comfrey, common dogwood, com-

mon self-heal, common yarrow, cork oak, crosswort, cypress, dandelion, dog rose, elm, hare's ear, hazel, horsetail, knotweed, labdanum,
medlar, mountain ash, mouse-ear hawkweed, myrtle, nettle, oak, periwinkle, plantain, pomegranate, puffball mushroom, quince, rose, small
cranberry, Solomon's seal, stonecrop, sumac, sweet chestnut, tormentil,
water caltrop, wintergreen, wood anemone, wood sanicle, wild carrot,
wild geranium, yellow iris.

Class 3.2. Detersive Vulneraries

Effects: heals and cicatrizes wounds and ulcers.

Plants: adder's tongue, bitter melon, blackberry, blue fenugreek,
buttercup, common ragwort, common soapwort, eggleaf twayblade, garlic mustard, greater celandine, gum copal, herb Barbara, honeysuckle,
ivy, nipplewort, old man's beard, prickly saltwort, privet, spotted lady's
thumb.

Class 3.3. Aperitive Vulneraries

Effects: provokes the appetite, unblocks obstructions, and clears
crude, sticky phlegm through the urine.

Plants: bastard balm, bugle, common speedwell, germander speedwell, golden marguerite, goldenrod, mountain arnica, rosin, Saint John's
wort, salad burnet.

Class 3.4. Emollients

Effects: relaxes and distends the tissues, muscles, and fibers, amelio-
rates mucous membranes, and soothes irritation.

Plants: bear's-breech, creeping toadflax, eastern pellitory-of-the-
wall, flax, Good King Henry, groundsel, holly, hogweed, lily, mallow,
marsh mallow, mercury, olive, orach, poplar, sea beet, spinach, violet.

Class 3.5. Resolutives for Topical Use

Effects: softens and breaks up tumors and dissolves coagulated or
fixed humors.

Plants: barley, bitter vetch, black bryony, buckwheat, common
figwort, common vetch, cotton thistle, dog figwort, enchanter's

nightshade, fava bean, fenugreek, field bindweed, hedge woundwort, lentil, lupine, marsh woundwort, oats, pea, rye, white wheat, wild woad.

Class 3.6. Calmatives and Soporifics
Effects: soothes pain and provokes sleep.
Plants: belladonna, bittersweet, eggplant, jimsonweed, hemlock, henbane, mandrake, opium poppy, tomato.

Class 3.7. Refreshing and Temperate Plants
Effects: tempers hot humors and refreshes the blood.
Plants: black currant, broadleaf plantain, cherry, chickweed, common duckweed, cucumber, currant, endive, gum arabic, hound's-tongue, houseleek, lamb's lettuce, lettuce, marsh pennywort, melon, mulberry, pine, proso millet, pumpkin, purslane, rice, romaine, raspberry, sow thistle, spiked rampion, tragacanth, water lily, willow.

3
Boerhaave's Classifications
of Medicinal Plants

T he following classifications, from which the herbal practitioner can profit considerably, have been compiled by the author from the writings of the Dutch botanist and chemist Herman Boerhaave (1668–1738), an admirably conscientious physician and scholar.[1]

Acidic, Sour, and Astringent Plants

Acacia, apple, ash bark, barberry, bistort root, bloody dock, caper fruit and root, cinquefoil, common houseleek, cypress fruit and leaves, dock, dog rose leaves and rosehips, dogwood leaves and green fruits, fern root, hypocist, green loquats, myrobalan, myrrh leaves, pomegranate, quince, rhubarb, Saint John's wort, salad burnet, sorb apple, sorrel, strawberry, sumac leaves and seeds, tamarind fruit, tamarisk bark, tomato, tormentil root, verjuice, white water lily leaves, wild plum, and almost all green fruits.

These plants should be prepared by infusion, by decoction, or with white wines by circulation.

Non-Acidic and Neutral Plants

Angelica, anise, arugula, asparagus, basil, blessed thistle, blue eryngo, cabbage, calamint, catnip, celery, clove, common agrimony, common centaury, common soapwort, cuckoopint, dill, elecampane, February daphne, garlic, garlic mustard, German chamomile, ginger, greater galangal, hedge mustard, horehound, horseradish, leek, long birth-wort, marjoram, milk thistle, mustard, nettle, onion, onionweed, oregano, pepper, pepper cress, pyrethrum, round-leaved birthwort, rue, satyrion, savin, savory, scurvy grass, squill, sweet flag, turnip, thyme, victory onion, watercress, white stonecrop, white swallow-wort, wild carrot, wild thyme, wormwood, yellow monkshood, zedoary.

These plants should be prepared in the same manner as the preceding group.

Alkaline Plants

Alyssum, arugula, bitter cress, black cumin, caper spurge, creeping gratiola, false flax, garlic mustard, germander, greater celandine, hedge mustard, motherwort, orpine, red pepper, spurge laurel, stinking goosefoot, watercress.

Refreshing Plants

Blackberry, citron, cucumber, elderberry, fig, jujube, lemon, muskmelon, orange, peach, pomegranate, raspberry, red currant, squash, strawberry, wild cherry.

Soothing and Emollient Plants

Artichoke, black cumin, black salsify root, borage, chervil, chicory, cucumber, dandelion, endive, goatsbeard root, lettuce, marsh valerian, orach, parsnip, purslane, rave, red cabbage, spinach, sweet almond, sweet potato, water parsnip root, and all floury cereals.

Mucilaginous and Demulcent Plants

Bear's-breech, black nightshade, black poplar leaves, chickweed, comfrey, creeping toadflax, daisy, eastern pellitory-of-the-wall, edelweiss, elderberry leaves, flax, Good King Henry, great mullein, henbane leaves, hound's-tongue, kidney vetch, lungwort, Madonna lily bulbs, marsh mallow (flowers, leaves, and roots), mercury, rose mallow (flowers, leaves, and roots), scabious, Solomon's seal, violet, wild mallow, white poplar leaves, yellow sweet clover.

Oily, Sweet, and Bitter Plants

Almond, flax, black nightshade, common comfrey, jujube, lichen, maidenhair spleenwort, mucilages, oil palm, olive, violet, white poppy, yellow sweet clover.

Aromatic and Cordial Plants

Anise, bay laurel, caraway, cinnamon, clove, fennel, geranium, hyssop, juniper, lavender, mace, marjoram, mint, nutmeg, oregano, pennyroyal, rosemary, saffron, sage, savory, thyme, wild thyme, wormwood.

From these aromatic plants the practitioner can draw essential balsamic oils of great virtue.

Irritant and Aromatic Plants Whose Flowers and Leaves Are Filled with Stimulant and Active Principles

Ageratum, anise, betony, birthwort, carnation, cat thyme, common agrimony, common centaury, dill, lavender, marigold, saffron, sage, scabious, southernwood, tansy, yellow sweet clover.

Aromatic Plants Whose Roots Contain Stimulant and Active Principles

Angelica, anise, benzoin, black alder, butcher's broom, butterbur, carline thistle, contrayerva, common restharrow, costmary, cyclamen, fennel, figwort, fraxinella, garlic, gentian, ginger, greater celandine, greater galangal, horseradish, iris, leopard's-bane, lovage, madder, nutsedge, parsley, peony, pyrethrum, round-leaved birthwort, satyrion, sea lavender, spignel, squill, sweet flag, turmeric, valerian, victory onion, wild angelica, white swallowwort, yellow monkshood, zedoary.

Aromatic or Stimulant Plants Whose Virtue Resides Chiefly in the Seed

Anise, arugula, bay laurel, burdock, caraway, cardamom, cashew, celery, columbine, common corn cockle, coriander, cubeb pepper, cumin, dill, fenugreek, hedge mustard, horseradish, juniper, kermes oak, lovage,

Massilian hartwort, mustard, nutmeg, parsley, parsnip, star anise, turnip, watercress, wild carrot, wild celery.

Plants Whose Virtue
Resides Chiefly in the Bark

Cinnamon, citron, guaiac wood, juniper, lemon, orange, sassafras.

Aromatic and Irritant Plant Saps

Aloin, liquid ambergris, asafetida, benzoin, frankincense, juniper, myrrh, sagapenum, storax.

Sudorific Plants Whose Virtue
Resides in the Roots

Black salsify, borage flowers, burdock, butcher's broom, chicory, couch grass, dandelion flowers, elderberry flowers, endive leaves, greenbrier, parsley, sarsaparilla, sorrel leaves, turnip, wild celery, wild turnip.

Diuretic and Detersive Plants

Artichoke, birch sap, butcher's broom, chervil, common hop, couch grass, dandelion, endive, lettuce, leek, parsley, sorrel, tea plant, wild chicory, and fresh-squeezed juices of ripe fruits.

Refreshing and Febrifugal Plants

Barberry, barley water, currant, lemon, mulberry, orange, pomegranate, quince, raspberry, wild cherry.

Hepatic Plants for Jaundice

Citron juice, dandelion, dock, endive, fumitory, grape, Good King Henry, hawkweed, lettuce, orange juice, prune, purslane, rush skeleton weed, silver cinquefoil, sorrel, tamarind, wild chicory, wood sorrel.

Plants for Intestinal Inflammation

Black salsify root, chicory root, goatsbeard root, lovage leaves, parsley root, Saint John's wort leaves, simarouba, valerian root, water parsnip root.

Antinephritic Plants

Agrimony, chervil, common bugloss, common restharrow, couch grass, creeping jenny, daisy, dandelion, eastern pellitory-of-the-wall, edelweiss, fennel, goldenrod, hairy rupturewort, hart's tongue fern, lettuce, licorice, marsh mallow, mercury, nettle, scabious, spotted lady's thumb, strawberry, vervain mallow, water lily, wild carrot.

Plant Oils for Paralysis
(for Topical Use)

Castor oil, catnip, chamomile, dill, iris, Persian clover, rue, saffron, wormwood.

All these oils may be blended together.

Antiscorbutic Plants

Agrimony, burdock, chervil, chickweed, chicory, common agrimony, dock, endive, fennel, fumitory, galega, garlic germander, germander, ground ivy, lemon balm, lovage, marjoram, mint, mugwort, nettle, sage, scabious, sea kale, sorrel, southernwood, speedwell, watercress, wood sorrel, yellow bugle, and all watery, acidulous, and sweet fruits.

Pulmonary Plants

Betony flowers, common poppy flowers, frankincense, licorice, myrrh, opium poppy, poppy seed, plantain, primrose, red cinquefoil flowers, Saint John's wort, silver cinquefoil, sorrel seed, tormentil root, turpentine tree.

Antiedemic Plants

Angelica root, bay laurel berries, birthwort root, cat thyme berries, common centaury flowers, fennel seeds, ginger root, juniper berries, laserwort root, rosemary flowers, tansy seeds, thyme berries, wild grape flowers, wild thyme berries, wormwood seeds, zedoary root.

These plants may be macerated together in strong aged wine.

Venereal Plants for Diseases
of the Womb and Ovaries

Asafetida, birthwort, bistort, cat thyme, chamomile, colocynth, elderberry, galbanum, juniper, marjoram, motherwort, mugwort, myrrh, pennyroyal, rue, sagapenum, sage, savin, tansy, thyme, wild thyme.

Plants for Resolving Bladder and Kidney Stones

Bear's-breech leaves, black salsify root, borage, chervil, eastern pellitory-of-the-wall leaves, goatsbeard root, lettuce, mallow leaves, marsh mallow leaves, mercury leaves, orach leaves, parsley, rose mallow leaves, rush skeleton weed, sow thistle root, water parsnip root, wild carrot root, wild turnip root.

Fortifying, Desiccant, Excitant, and Stimulant Plants

Agrimony, angelica, betony, blackberry, caper berries, carline thistle, cashew, clove, dodder, great golden maidenhair, hart's tongue fern, lemon balm, liverwort, male fern, polypody, royal fern, rustyback, sandalwood, scabious, speedwell, squill, tamarisk, wood sanicle.

4

Methods of
Plant Preservation

To a certain extent this issue falls outside the scope of our investigation. To be sure, there is no shortage of works that cover the subject in great detail, but it would be beneficial here to draw the reader's attention to a few of the finer points.

During their growth, plants accumulate a viscous water that becomes an integral part of their constitution. But they are also saturated with a raw, undeveloped, and superabundant water that must be separated from their substance because it causes their corruption. It should be obvious to readers that this is particularly necessary for plants of Ettmüller's 1st Class, which are filled with this tasteless water. It is therefore necessary to proceed by desiccation, and various heat sources may be employed to this end, such as the heat of the Sun, the drying stove, the bain-marie, or the special oven. These means of desiccation may be employed separately or successively depending on the particular nature of the plant.

Take wild chicory, for example, which contains a moderate proportion of this raw water. First separate the foreign weeds and dead leaves, then spread out the fresh leaves on small wicker racks covered with parchment paper and expose them to the heat of the Sun or put them in a special oven at an average temperature of 100 or 125 degrees Fahrenheit. You will know the plant has finished drying when it pulverizes to the touch. Remove it from the oven and expose it to the air in a clean, shady, and dry place, ensuring that the leaves and stems are not piled on top of each other. When prepared in this manner, plants retain their color and fresh appearance.

Aromatic plants must be dried *as quickly as possible,* but the heat must be proportioned to the degree of volatility of their spirit or spirituous salt and their quantity of moisture. In this case, exposure to the heat of the Sun is preferable to the bain-marie. Some plants that are used fresh-picked should not be dried, because their virtue resides in their juices and volatile salts, which dissipate under heat. The same is true of the cruciferous and antiscorbutic plants. For other plants it seems that their aroma diminishes after desiccation, but this is only apparent, because their scent or perfume reappears gradually.

Fruits

Fruits, berries, grains, seeds, stones, and pips are one and the same thing but differently constituted, for the seed is always at the center of the fruit. The seed contains the germ of the plant, and it forms only after flowering, at the time of maturity.

Whatever fruit you wish to dry should be harvested *before* it is fully ripe, but any fruit you wish to use immediately should be picked when it is ripe, tasty, sweet, and colorful. Peel the fruits and heat them in the oven for a quarter of an hour. Remove them and expose them to the air or to the Sun until the process of desiccation is almost complete. Then separate them from each other with parchment paper and dry them with a slow heat (*ignis lentus*).

Flowers

All parts of the flower are not equally fragrant, nor is the flower always the seat of the scent. Among Lamiaceae such as thyme, rosemary, sage, and lavender, the odor resides in the calyx, but the leaves of these plants have just as much odor as their flowers and provide equal amounts of essential oil in distillation. Among Liliaceae such as white lilies, yellow lilies, tulips, and plants of the jasmine and orange blossom species, the odor emanates from the petals. These flowers, as well as most pale roses, should be used fresh, as they lose their fragrance after desiccation. The fragrance of these flowers is so fleeting that it can only be retained by their oily principle. Other flowers like red roses, red carnations, and white mullein acquire odor through desiccation.

The best time to pick flowers is just before they blossom, although there are a few rare exceptions to this rule. Red carnation and sweet violet should be gathered the moment the flower blossoms. The same is true for some very small flowers such as common centaury, garlic germander, wormwood, hyssop, fumitory, marjoram, oregano, sweet-scented bedstraw, and yellow bedstraw, whose flowering tops should be preserved. Chamomile flowers should be cut from their stems, and coltsfoot and catsfoot flowers need to be dried longer than others. In short, the process of desiccation for flowers is analogous to that for both plants and leaves: they are preserved in the same manner. As a general rule, it is best to leave them their calyx to aid in their preservation.

Seeds

Oily seeds or almonds that are emulsive such as flax, citron, psyllium, sweet and bitter almonds, melon, cucumber, cumin, anise, and fennel yield their oil by expression after they have been dried in the autumn Sun in an arid place. Remove their shell and leave them their yellow and tender pulp. If there is no sunlight, the bain-marie is a desideratum. In floury seeds such as barley, oats, rye, lupines, peas, lentils, kidney beans, and fava beans, the mucilage is desiccated and can be dissolved only in boiling water.

Dry and fine seeds like those of coriander and wormseed are difficult to pulverize. Gather them together with their stem and dry them in the Sun. Then merely shake the stem and the seeds will fall off. Expose them to the air for two days and preserve them in sealed glass jars.

Roots

We shall speak later about the best time to pick certain roots as this is a subject on which there is much disagreement, but bulbous or oily roots can be gathered in any season. To preserve the roots, first wash them with fresh water, then cut them into pieces and dry them in the oven. They should then be stored in tightly sealed tin boxes.

Some roots such as marsh mallow and water lily do not keep for very long. Angelica root is best harvested in spring, as it does not keep for as long when it has been harvested in autumn.

Woods

Woods should be harvested in autumn after the leaves have fallen. Large branches should be taken along with the bark, except for juniper wood, whose bark and sapwood is to be discarded.

Exotic softwoods such as aloeswood and guaiac wood must be selected when they are compact and heavy, without sapwood, and especially from the area around the trunk. Cut the wood into pieces after removing as much of their bark and sapwood as possible, then dry them on the underside of the wood. Softwoods can be stored for long periods of time, but they need to be kept in well-sealed tin boxes and stored in a dry place. Barks can be dried and preserved in the same manner as woods, but it is necessary to wash them thoroughly beforehand.

The Vallot Method of Plant Preservation

Harvest the plant between flower and seed at sunrise and in dry weather. Stack them in large sandstone containers and pack them in until the containers are filled to the brim. Insert stoppers previously dipped in melted wax into the necks of the containers and then coat the tops of the stoppers with melted pitch.[1] This method works extremely well and will preserve plants for long periods of time without losing their virtue, fragrance, or flavor. Moreover, they will ferment themselves and thus be well prepped for future distillations.*

N.B.: A pinch of raw salt niter placed in the bottom of the container produces an excellent effect.

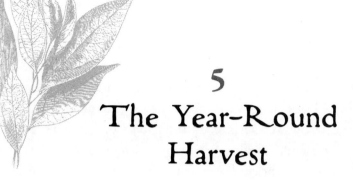

5
The Year-Round
Harvest

March (♓–♈)

Flowers: lily bulbs, peach blossom, periwinkle, primrose.

Roots: arum, asparagus, birthwort, bistort, black hellebore, bryony, burdock, butcher's broom, cinquefoil, common reed, couch grass, cyclamen, dropwort, fennel, figwort, greater celandine, iris, male fern, restharrow, satyrion, saxifrage, sorrel, sweet flag, tormentil, water lily, white hellebore, wild celery.

April (♈–♉)

Anything that was not harvested in March due to bad weather should be harvested in April, in addition to the following: dock root, field marigold flowers, lily of the valley flowers, mandrake leaves, rose bedeguar gall, walnut catkins, white nettle flowers, wild chicory root.

May (♉–♊)

Anything that was not harvested in April due to inclement weather should be harvested in May, the month when vegetation is most active and abundant, in addition to the following: agrimony, borage, broom flowers, bugle, chamomile flowers, common agrimony, common bugloss, common hop, elderberry bark and flowers, fumitory flowers, geranium flowers, German chamomile, ground ivy, hemlock, lungwort, mercury, peony flowers, periwinkle, plantain, white and red rose flowers, rue, scabious, sea wormwood, speedwell, tansy, turnip seeds, wild chicory, wormwood, and all antiscorbutic plants.

June (♊–♋)

Harvest almost all May plants when they are late, in addition to angelica, basil, betony, black horehound, black nightshade, blessed thistle, calamint, caraway seeds, cherries, clary sage, common centaury, common soapwort, coriander seeds, currants, dandelion, dill, edelweiss, European wild ginger, eyebright leaves, fennel leaves, flax-leaved daphne bark, garlic germander, henbane, hyssop, lemon balm leaves, lesser dodder, mallow leaves, marjoram, marsh mallow leaves, mugwort, oregano, peppermint, sage, strawberries, sundew, thyme seeds, tobacco, wall germander, white horehound, wild celery, wormseed wallflower leaves, yellow bedstraw, yellow sweet clover.

Flowers: borage, common bugloss, common poppy, cornflower, French lavender, lavender, linden, Madonna lily, mallow, marsh mallow, musk rose, orange blossom, pussytoe, Saint John's wort, scabious, sneezewort, white mullein.

July (♋–♌)

Harvest all late aromatic plants in addition to black currant, black cherries, mulberries, opium poppy heads, raspberries, sumac, green (unripe) walnuts.

Leaves: cat thyme, common yarrow, creeping gratiola, figwort, greater celandine, groundsel, hoary stock, lesser catmint, meadowsweet, savin, spotted lady's thumb, wood sanicle.

Seeds: dill, bitter vetch, black poppy, field pennycress, hartwort, lupine, parsley, psyllium, violet, wild carrot.

August (♌–♍)

August is the month of maturity. Harvest belladonna leaves, bog bean leaves, cucumber seeds, henbane seeds, hairy rupturewort leaves, jimsonweed, muskmelon seeds, pomegranate blossoms, rosehips, wild carrot seeds.

September (♍–♎)

Angelica root, autumn crocus root, barberries, buckthorn berries, Chinese lantern berries, elderberries, hart's tongue fern, licorice root, maidenhair fern, maidenhair spleenwort, muskmelon seeds, nettle seeds, orchis root, pumpkin seeds, rustyback, valerian root.

October (♎–♏)

Castor oil seeds, common mistletoe, coriander seeds, flax-leaved daphne bark, golden reinette apple, juniper wood and berries, peony seeds, quince, red cabbage, sumac.

Roots: angelica, blue eryngo, common comfrey, dock, elecampane, hound's-tongue, madder, polypody, potato, purple star thistle, rhapontic rhubarb, rhubarb, wild angelica.

November (♏–♐)

Remaining vegetation, agaric, juniper berries, some mushrooms.

December (♐–♑)

December is the month of atony. It is best to rest during this period of time.

January (♑–♒)

Cypress nuts, tree lungwort.

February (♒–♓)

Buds: coltsfoot, poplar, violet, wallflower.

Roots: European wild ginger, marsh mallow, parsley, peony, polypody, strawberry, valerian, yellow monkshood.

Ancient Groupings of Plants with Common Properties

- **The five aperitive roots:** butcher's broom, asparagus, fennel, parsley, and wild celery.
- **The five capillaries:** Southern maidenhair fern, black spleenwort, great golden maidenhair, rustyback (or, in its place, hart's tongue fern), and wall rue.

🖋 **The three cordial flowers:** common bugloss, borage, and violet.

🖋 **The four carminative flowers:** Roman chamomile, yellow sweet clover, German chamomile, and dill.

🖋 **The common emollient herbs:** mallow leaves, marsh mallow leaves, bear's-breech leaves, violet leaves, mercury leaves, eastern pellitory-of-the-wall leaves, beet leaves, groundsel leaves, and lily bulbs.

🖋 **The four greater cold seeds:** squash, pumpkin, melon, and cucumber.

🖋 **The four lesser cold seeds:** lettuce, purslane, endive, and chicory.

🖋 **The four greater hot seeds:** anise, fennel, caraway, and cumin, which are also called carminatives.

🖋 **The four lesser hot seeds:** wild celery, parsley, bishop's weed, and wild carrot.

Conventional Aphorisms of the Ancients

The preceding classifications are for the most part based on the effects produced in the human body by plants that have been prepared in a basic manner according to the processes of ordinary chemistry. The properties indicated in these classifications thus pertain to allopathic medicine, which seeks to cure an illness by its opposite according to the aphorism of antipathy, *contraria contrariis curantur* or "opposites are cured by opposites." However, the situation is quite different with respect to *astral correspondences* because these proceed from spagyric medicine (from which the science of modern homeopathy was born), which seeks to cure an illness by its like according to the aphorism of sympathy, *similia similibus curantur* or "likes are cured by likes."

Any plant, in fact, with few exceptions, that has been treated by ordinary processes will act in a basic, innocuous, and superficial manner. However, when the same plant has been treated by spagyric processes, in other words, when the quintessence has been extracted from the plant, its action alters drastically and it will operate in a much more profound manner: it will destroy the source of an illness by means of a natural principle that resembles its source.

We shall cover in due course the various methods of preparing plants according to the ordinary chemical procedures of the most accomplished premodern chemists. First, however, it is necessary to discuss a subject which the masters of spagyric chemistry have always considered to be of capital importance, namely the appropriate annual and astral times for harvesting medicinal plants.

Determining the Best Times of Year to Harvest Medicinal Plants

All years are not equally favorable for harvesting plants. The best years are those with moderate rainfall. Dry years are good for harvesting plants of a hot and aromatic nature such as angelica, thyme, juniper, anise, clove, pepper, and mint, as their essential principles possess less virtue in rainy years, which are less favorable both to plant growth and to plant preservation.

Perennials are fortified by the Universal Spirit at the vernal and autumnal equinoxes, and for this reason it is best to harvest them from the first days of April, whereas their roots are best harvested at the beginning of October when they are saturated with the essential principles that constitute their virtue. Annuals, on the other hand, are not preserved by their roots and their virtue varies *according to the stage of their growth at the time of harvest.* Thus, borages in the first stages of their growth contain very small quantities of earthy alkali salt and niter, but as their growth progresses the quantity of these salts gradually increases. Crucifers and most annual aromatics are subject to the same natural laws.

Almost all authors agree that plants should be harvested just when their buds are beginning to open or just before the flower opens or blooms, in other words, *between flower and seed.* This is especially true for species of calamint, centaury, bugle, germander, fumitory, marjoram, oregano, pennyroyal, thyme, and wild thyme. However, the between-flower-and-seed rule is by no means absolute. Certain aqueous plants such as lettuce and romaine and soothing and lenitive plants like mallow, marsh mallow, eastern pellitory-of-the-wall, and groundsel possess dulcifying and salutary principles only when they are young, that is, before their stems shoot up. The same is true of chicory, species of cabbage, common agrimony, plantain, and various species of dock, as their leaves become woody after their stems shoot up. Plants whose virtue resides in their fruits or berries should be harvested only when they are very ripe so that their fruits or seeds have had time to form. Some plants produce only tiny embryonic flowers such as maidenhair ferns, hart's tongue fern, and polypody. The fructifying principles of these plants are contained in the cottony down that garnishes the underside of their leaves when they have fully matured.

The dogbane, among other plants, provides ample proof of the kinds of modifications that occur in the nature of plants at the different stages of their growth, since it is well known that this plant is salutary in its youth but becomes poisonous when it is ripe. Similarly, the young sprouts of the elderberry are much more purgative than its mature leaves. *It is therefore necessary to know the nature of a plant at the various stages of its formation.* Some writers suggest that seeds should be harvested when the plant is very ripe, well nourished, full, fragrant, and strong in flavor. Others say that seeds should be harvested before they become too ripe, that is, before their vital principle or mercurial moisture dissipates. What is certain is that the scent and the taste of seeds are signs of their perfection, but for inodorous and insipid seeds it is much more difficult to determine the perfect times to harvest them. On this matter Le Fèvre says that it is necessary to harvest them before the wet mercurial essence that is their vital principle weakens.[1]

The harvesting of roots should be performed when the stems are spent, dry, or faded, which usually takes place in the fall or in the spring. But authors disagree when it comes to choosing one or the other season. Dioscorides, Galen, and Avicenna suggest that the best time is at the beginning of winter, when the leaves have begun to fall, because, they say, when the plant dries out, its sap recedes into the roots, which remain alive in the earth and ready to vegetate anew, as is the case with succulent or bulbous plants. On the other hand, Marcello Malpighi and several others claim that the "winter numbness" of plants is only apparent and that they continue to vegetate in the ground. Proponents of this view suggest that roots—with the exception of bulbous roots, which are good in all seasons—should be harvested when their leaf packs start to emerge from the ground, because the winter cold preserves the sap secreted by the roots in autumn, which develops in the spring and breathes new life into the roots. In the spring, roots are full, fleshy, and succulent, whereas in autumn they are exhausted from supplying juice to the plant over the course of the summer and become hard and woody.

Obviously, the question is not an easy one to answer. Some expert practitioners suggest that autumn roots are best for the purposes of preservation and desiccation, because spring roots abound in insipid watery principles that are lacking in virtue. According to Boerhaave, spring roots are weak and devoid of vigor because they are at the beginning stages of their growth and their saps are watery, immature, and deficient in essential, resinous, and saline principles. The excess water, furthermore, makes them susceptible to fermentation when they are laid out to dry. This proves, as Antoine Baumé maintains, that succulence is not a prerequisite for harvesting roots, and this is an opinion we share.[2]

Several authors recommend picking plants a little after sunrise, so that the dew water with which they are saturated has had time to evaporate. But Paracelsus and his school say that the best time is a little before sunrise, when plants are saturated with Universal Spirit and dew water, which awakens and exalts their virtue. Paracelsus calls this temporal period *balsamiticum tempus* or "balsamic time." Be that as it may, we advise the practitioner to adopt the first opinion only for leafy, tender, and watery plants like lettuce, lamb's lettuce, romaine, chicory, and all salads in general. In all cases, it is essential that the weather be clear and serene at the time of harvest.

Determining Under What Astral Influences to Harvest Medicinal Plants

The Moon exerts a profound influence on plants as well as on the humors of the human body. It is therefore necessary to understand the nature of its influences, in parallel with those of the Sun, when harvesting plants.

The most favorable lunar position is when the Moon is ascending and three days before it is full. Harvests should be avoided when the Moon is descending or when it is conjoined, opposed, or squared by the Sun.* Favorable aspects are when the Moon is in sextile or trine to the Sun.

---

*The ascending quadrature (first quarter), being of a generous nature (hot and wet), does not have the maleficent character of the descending quadrature (last quarter), which is cold and dry.

Some authors recommend picking a plant when its ruling planet is in a good aspect to the Sun and the Moon. Others suggest that the plant's ruling planet or one of the zodiacal signs corresponding to the plant should be either at the Ascendant or at the Upper Meridian. Still others prefer to have Jupiter or Venus in a good aspect to the plant's ruling planet or at least in one of the plant's corresponding zodiacal signs. It is always beneficial when one of the plant's ruling planets is in one of the plant's corresponding zodiacal signs, if, that is, it is not otherwise unfavorably aspected. (The correspondences of plants to the planets and zodiacal signs are provided at the beginning of the next chapter.)

All this may seem hopelessly complex, but we believe it is necessary first to determine the position of the Moon and its aspect to the Sun, and then to determine whether it is possible to combine this relationship with any other favorable influences. However, one must never operate when the luminaries (the Sun and the Moon) are negatively aspected to each other or when they receive unfavorable rays from Mars or Saturn, or even, some say, from Neptune and Uranus. With a little discernment it should be easy to fix the appropriate times for plant harvests, which practitioners can determine well in advance with the aid of an ephemeris.

Determining Under What Astral Influences to Administer Herbal Remedies

Rule 1. The luminaries must be in a good aspect to each other or to Jupiter and Venus, and they must not be negatively aspected by maleficent rays from Mars and Saturn.

Rule 2. The point of the Ascendant in the patient's birth chart must not be affected by malefics.

Rule 3. The luminaries must not be in houses VI, VIII, or XII of the patient's birth chart.

One must also take into account the patient's temperament in the administration of remedies, for if the temperament is sanguine, the cure must be administered at sunrise; if choleric, at noon; if phlegmatic, at midnight; and if melancholic, at sunset (see Table 1.1 on page 16).*

---

*If the patient's temperament is mixed, it is necessary to administer the remedy at whatever time corresponds to the mean between the two respective joint positions.

Some also suggest that the patient's Sun sign should be found at the Ascendant (Asc) or at Midheaven (MC). Others prefer that the most beneficent planet in the subject's birth chart be in a positive aspect to one of the luminaries. The Moon in trine to the Sun or Jupiter is always favorable, if they are not otherwise negatively aspected.

If for some reason it is not possible to draw up the patient's birth chart, it suffices to observe *Rule 1*.

6

Plant Signatures

Correspondences of Plants to the Planets and the Signs of the Zodiac

The simple and mixed bodies of creation all participate in the combined natures of the Sun, the Moon, and the planets in various proportions. The influence of the planets on plants is never isolated, because their influx acts in concert and in a permanent way, but the nature and power of their radiation varies according to their aspects and positions. Hence, one may assume that the particular nature of a given plant is rarely analogous to that of a single planet and, moreover, that each plant participates in the natures of all the planets combined, but in varying proportions.[1]

There are several modes of correspondence. Some are based on analogies of character and constitution such as form, appearance, growth, substance, color, scent, and taste, while others are based on analogies between the spirit or soul of the plant and the intimate nature of the planet. The first mode relates to the generative nature of the stars, the second to their action on the human body. We adopt the second mode of correspondence, which, in any case, is often in harmony with the first.[2]

This classification is divisible into as many groups as there are planets, the Sun and the Moon included. The planetary and zodiacal signs following the plant names listed below represent influences of secondary nature, according to which the herbal practitioner can distinguish the specific nature of each plant belonging to a given planetary group.

The quintessences of these plants must be prescribed and administered after the completion of thorough and comparative examinations first of the patient and then of the patient's birth chart. When the practitioner has acquired knowledge of the intimate nature of the illness, he or she should then consult the analogical correspondences of the planets with the organic functions of the human body provided in chapter 11 and in this manner determine the planetary nature of the disease. This will enable the practitioner to select a plant that has an identical astral nature. The quintessence of the plant administered will cure the illness "by its like" according to the aphorism of sympathy: *similia similibus curantur.*

Plants Ruled by the Sun (☉)

Angelica: ♀ ♌ ♋
Chamomile: ☿ ♀ ♌ ♊ ♉ ♋
Cinnamon: ♀ ♃ ♋ ♍ ♎
Eyebright: ☾ ♂ ♌ ♋ ♏
Greater Celandine: ♂ ♄ ♌ ♈ ♋
Hyssop: ♃ ♈ ♎ ♐
Knotweed: ♃ ♊ ♐
Mountain Arnica: ♂ ♄ ♌ ♈ ♒
Nutmeg: ♂ ♃ ♊ ♐ ♌
Peppermint: ♂ ♀ ♍ ♎ ♏
Pinkroot: ☿ ♌ ♈ ♊
Rosemary: ♃ ♊ ♎ ♓
Sage: ♂ ♃ ♈ ♍ ♐
Scarlet Pimpernel: ☿ ♍
Speedwell: ♂ ☿ ♈ ♌ ♍
Thyme: ☿ ♊ ♋ ♍

Plants Ruled by the Moon (☾)

Bhilawa: ♂ ♋ ♈
Bittersweet: ♄ ♀ ♑ ♉ ♏
Black Cohosh: ☿ ♏ ♑
Cactus: ♀ ♂ ♏ ♎ ♋
Colocynth: ♂ ♀ ♏ ♎
Common Poppy: ☿ ♉ ♊
Cucumber: ♓ ♋
Curly Dock: ♀ ♉ ♒ ♊
Fool's Parsley: ☿ ♓ ♍
Hemlock: ♄ ♋ ♏ ♒
Horsetail: ♄ ♑ ♓
Ipecacuanha: ☉ ♉ ♋
Iris: ♂ ♓ ♈
Jalap: ♋ ♍ ♏
Parsley: ♂ ♓ ♈
Poison Ivy: ♄ ☉ ♈ ♑ ♐
Purging Croton: ♂ ♑ ♏
Rhatany: ♀ ♓ ♏ ♉
Rhubarb: ♄ ♋ ♑
Rockrose: ♀ ♄ ♉ ♑
Watercress: ♃ ♉ ♋ ♍
Water Hemlock: ♀ ♑ ♓

Plants Ruled by Saturn (♄)

Asafetida: ♀ ♂ ♑ ♎ ♏

Belladonna: ☿ ♎ ♍ ♋ ♑

Black Hellebore: ☿ ☾ ♎ ♑ ♏

Buttercup: ☿ ☉ ♌ ♒ ♍

Common Soapwort: ♀ ♎ ♑

Indian Hemp: ♀ ☿ ♉ ♊ ♒

Monkshood: ♂ ☉ ☿ ♌ ♈ ♍ ♒

Sarsaparilla: ♀ ♃ ♉ ♊ ♒

Plants Ruled by Jupiter (♃)

Agrimony: ☿ ♉ ♍

Ammoniacum: ♄ ♌ ♍

Bay Laurel: ☉ ♈ ♌ ♐

Birch: ☿ ♍ ♏ ♎

Borage: ♀ ♈ ♌ ♐

Cedar: ☉ ♄ ♌ ♒ ♊

Centaury: ☉ ♌ ♏ ♎

Chervil: ☿ ♊ ♉ ♐

Endive: ☾ ♉ ♋ ♓

Eucalyptus: ♊ ♌ ♐

Henbane: ♄ ♋ ♒ ♐

Lemon Balm: ☉ ♌ ♋ ♍

Linden: ☾ ♊ ♉ ♐

Maritime Squill: ☾ ♓ ♋

Red Trillium: ♀ ♊ ♉ ♓

Savin: ♀ ☿ ♐ ♍ ♎

Plants Ruled by Mars (♂)

Aloe: ♀ ♄ ♑ ♏ ♎

Autumn Crocus: ♄ ♏ ♑

Blessed Thistle: ♃ ♉ ♊ ♍

Bryony: ☿ ♈ ♊ ♋ ♌

Clematis: ☾ ♈ ♋

Common Boneset: ☾ ♑ ♉

Common Hop: ☿ ♋ ♍ ♏

Culver's Root: ☾ ♏ ♍ ♌

Ergot Fungus: ♀ ☿ ♍ ♎ ♏

Foxglove: ☿ ☾ ♈ ♌ ♋

Garlic: ♀ ♈ ♎

Gentian: ♋ ♌ ♍

Licebane: ♀ ♎ ♏ ♉

Mugwort: ☉ ♍ ♎ ♏

Purple Boneset: ♄ ♑ ♒

Quinine: ♄ ♉ ♏

Spurge: ☾ ♄ ♑ ♏

Strychnine Tree: ♀ ♏ ♍ ♌

Witch Hazel: ♃ ♈ ♏

Wormwood: ☉ ♈ ♌ ♐

Plants Ruled by Venus (♀)

Chaste Tree: ♄ ♏ ♉ ♍

Benzoin (flowers): ♊ ♉ ♐

Barberry: ♂ ♉ ♏

Cyclamen: ☉ ♉ ♌

False Unicorn (root): ♂ ♑ ♒ ♈

Figwort: ♉ ♋

Golden Ragwort: ☿ ♊ ♉

Jasmine: ☉ ♈ ♍

Marsh Mallow: ♉ ♊ ♋

Mayapple: ♂ ☾ ♎ ♏ ♑

Peony: ☉ ☾ ♋ ♎

Pasqueflower: ☿ ♂ ♈ ♋ ♊ ♏

Plantain: ☿ ♂ ♉ ♊ ♏

Pokeweed: ☿ ♂ ♈ ♍

Rhododendron: ♄ ♎ ♑ ♉

Senna: ☾ ♓

Vervain: ☿ ♊ ♍

Plants Ruled by Mercury (☿)

Agaric: ☾ ♂ ♍ ♉ ♈

Bindweed: ♀ ♊ ♒

Bloody Geranium: ♀ ☉ ♒ ♓

Burdock: ♀ ♎ ♏

Calabar Bean: ☾ ♂ ♍ ♏

Clover: ♀ ♓

Club Moss: ☾ ☉ ♈ ♓ ♋ ♏

Coffee: ♀ ♍ ♈

Eastern Pellitory-of-the-Wall: ♄ ♒

Elderberry: ☾ ♊ ♋ ♐

Fennel: ♑ ♉ ♐

Gelsemium: ♄ ♊ ♍ ♎

Ignatia: ♄ ♂ ♊ ♈ ♍ ♏

Lily of the Valley: ♀ ♊ ♐

Lungwort: ♉ ♋ ♐

Maidenhair Spleenwort: ♂ ♈ ♋

Mercury: ♊ ♍ ♒

Oats: ♀ ♋

Oregano: ☉ ♐

Primrose: ♀ ♈

Rue: ♀ ♄ ♒ ♍ ♎

Saint John's Wort: ☉ ☾ ♋ ♑ ♍

Savory: ☉ ♀ ♓ ♏

Scabious: ♀

Southernwood: ♀ ♍ ♎

Star Anise: ☉ ♉ ♋ ♏

Sundew: ☾ ♂ ♊ ♋

Tea Plant: ♉ ♊ ♐ ♍

Valerian: ♊ ♈ ♒

White Hellebore: ☾ ♂ ♈ ♉ ♋

Several modern homeopathic authors prescribe the following herbal medicines for diseases born of the four humoral temperaments:

1. *Sanguine temperament:* monkshood, mountain arnica, agaric, belladonna, bryony, white hellebore, strychnine tree, and pasqueflower.
2. *Choleric temperament:* bryony, black hellebore, greater celandine, club moss, culver's root, bloody geranium, and quinine.
3. *Phlegmatic temperament:* asafetida, belladonna, hemlock, ipecacuanha, and pasqueflower.
4. *Melancholic temperament:* monkshood, chamomile, coffee, Levant berry, water hemlock, gelsemium, ignatia, pinkroot, lily, and white hellebore.

The onus of responsibility for such generic treatments we leave on the shoulders of such authors.

Paracelsus asserts that not all plants are capable of giving a true quintessence, but he distinguishes two plants in particular whose quintessences are richest in virtue: *greater celandine* and *lemon balm*.

However, he also maintains that several other plants can approximate the nature of these two perfect specimens, such as common figwort and common centaury, among other vulneraries like wintergreen, common comfrey, goldenrod, Saint John's wort, wormwood, and almost all alexitaries such as garlic germander, gentian, rue, parsley, wild celery, and many others. We are of the opinion, however, that the virtue of any plant, no matter how great or small, can always be exalted spagyrically, and that if among plants of the same nature the practitioner comes to esteem some more than others for their excellence, then he or she may use them preferentially, for every cure depends on the value judgments of the one treating the illness.

The following are some of the more practical value judgments of the French astrologer Claude Dariot, who is perhaps best known for his translation of Paracelsus's *Der grossen Wundartzney* or *Great Surgery Book:* Peony root harvested when the Moon is conjoined with the Sun and hung around a patient's neck cures epilepsy. Woods cut when the Moon is full will rot. Purging should be avoided when the Moon is in Capricorn or Taurus. Vulneraries for stomach illnesses should be harvested when Virgo is at the Ascendant. In general, herbs should be gathered when they are in bloom and when the sign presiding over the organ the herb heals is at the Ascendant or at Midheaven. Lemon balm is the model for aromatic cordials, which are comforting and act against cold and wet humors. The following plants imitate its nature:

1. Fruits: juniper, ivy, bay laurel.
2. Seeds: anise, star anise, fennel, cumin, parsley.
3. Barks: orange, lemon, citron, mace, cinnamon.
4. Spices: nutmeg, clove, grains of paradise, cardamom, pepper, cubeb pepper.

Essence of cinnamon with water of mugwort, pennyroyal, or hyssop is good for women in labor. Clove is hot and dry and good for cold and wet ailments that affect the stomach, the heart, the womb, and the spleen, and for melancholic diseases. Mace is good for the stomach; pepper for cold colic and fever; and anise, fennel, and cumin are vermifugal and fortifying herbs that drive away melancholy. Juniper is good for the kidneys and kidney stones as well as the chest, hysteria, convulsions, paralysis, the nerves, the mind, and the bladder. Sage, rosemary, and lavender calm the mind. Savin, mugwort, and pennyroyal are good for menstrual cramps. To calm all body pains, grind dwarf elder seed, put it in a large vessel, pour eight fingers of water over it, and boil it for an hour while periodically removing the foam. Then put the material in a closed vessel and apply a very soft heat. When the oil ascends, separate it from the water. Rectify this oil by distillation, with four times as much fountain water, in the ash bath. This oil is intended for topical use.[3]

Determining the Times When the Sun and the Signs of the Zodiac Pass through the Four Angles

To aid practitioners in the harvesting of medicinal plants, we offer here a very simple procedure for determining the times of sunrise and sunset over the course of the year as well as the passage of the signs of the zodiac through the four astrological angles (for the provinces of France).

First of all, the Sun is always at the Upper Meridian or Midheaven (MC) in any location at noon, and so it will occupy the Lower Meridian or Nadir (IC) of the same place at midnight. Only the times of sunrise and sunset vary little by little each day, but with the aid of the annual table below, these variations are easy to determine. Table 6.1 on page 49 shows the places occupied by the Sun in the zodiac at the times of its rising and setting in ten-day intervals.

To calculate the astrological position of the Sun on a day that falls between two of these intervals, merely advance the Sun in the order of signs one degree per day from the first of the two intervals. For example, if one wishes to know the radical position the Sun will occupy on April 5, start at the indicator for April 1, when the Sun is at 10 degrees Aries, and add five degrees (one per day) to the degree indicator, which places the Sun at 15 degrees Aries on April 5.

The same procedure may be utilized to determine the hours of sunrise and sunset. From April 1 to April 10 the sunrise retrogrades 20 minutes (from 5:40 a.m. to 5:20 a.m.). To determine the time when the Sun will rise on April 5, between April 1 (5:40 am) and April 10 (5:20 a.m.), take one-half of the time retrograded (10 minutes) and subtract it from the preceding interval (5:40 a.m.), which gives 5:30 a.m. for the time of sunrise on April 5. This same procedure may also be used to determine the time of sunset, which occurs at 6:35 p.m. on April 5.

To determine the time when a zodiacal sign will pass over one of the four astrological angles, the procedure is equally simple. The zodiacal degree of the Sun must be taken from the table for the chosen day. This degree is invariable over the course of a single day, which means that the Sun will be at the same degree at sunrise, noon, sunset, and midnight. Once you know the zodiacal degree of the Sun for the day in question, take the time at which the Sun passes the chosen angle and count fifteen degrees per hour from the degree of the Sun, because the zodiac appears to traverse the sky from east to west at 30 degrees (an entire sign) in two hours' time. If, then, the Sun at noon (Upper Meridian) is in the 10th degree of Taurus, one hour later the 25th degree of the same sign will pass to the Upper Meridian, and two hours later the 10th degree of the next sign (Gemini) will occupy the Upper Meridian, and so on.*

---

*The point on the horizon where the Sun rises is called the Ascendant (Asc). The point perpendicular to the plane of the horizon where the Sun is at noon is called the Upper Meridian, Midheaven, or *Medium Coeli* (MC). The point on the horizon where the Sun sets is called the Descendant (Dsc). The point opposite the Upper Meridian, which the Sun occupies at midnight, is called the Nadir or *Imum Coeli* (IC).

TABLE 6.I.
CALCULATIONS OF SUNRISE AND SUNSET TIMES*

Sign	Degree	Month Day	Rising (AM)	Setting (PM)	Sign	Degree	Month Day	Rising (AM)	Setting (PM)
♈	0°	March 20	6:00	6:15	♎	0°	Sept. 23	5:50	6:00
	10°	April 1	5:40	6:30		10°	Oct. 1	6:00	5:40
	20°	April 10	5:20	6:40		20°	Oct. 11	6:15	5:20
♉	0°	April 20	5:00	7:00	♏	0°	Oct. 23	6:30	5:00
	10°	May 1	4:40	7:15		10°	Nov. 1	6:50	4:40
	20°	May 10	4:30	7:30		20°	Nov. 11	7:00	4:30
♊	0°	May 21	4:15	7:40	♐	0°	Nov. 22	7:20	4:15
	10°	June 1	4:00	7:50		10°	Dec. 1	7:30	4:00
	20°	June 10	4:00	8:00		20°	Dec. 10	7:40	4:00
♋	0°	June 21	4:00	8:00	♑	0°	Dec. 21	7:50	4:00
	10°	July 1	4:00	8:00		10°	Jan. 1	8:00	4:10
	20°	July 11	4:10	8:00		20°	Jan. 10	7:50	4:20
♌	0°	July 21	4:20	7:50	♒	0°	Jan. 20	7:40	4:30
	10°	August 1	4:35	7:30		10°	Feb. 1	7:30	4:50
	20°	August 11	4:50	7:20		20°	Feb. 9	7:20	5:10
♍	0°	August 23	5:00	7:00	♓	0°	Feb. 18	7:00	5:20
	10°	Sept. 1	5:20	6:40		10°	March 1	6:40	5:40
	20°	Sept. 11	5:30	6:20		20°	March 10	6:30	6:00

---

*[Mavéric was fond of inventing quick and simple procedures for calculating a variety of astrological phenomena. See especially his *La clef de l'horoscope quotidien*. Several of these dates are no longer precise, if indeed they were ever intended to be. Mavéric calculates all subsequent dates in this book, e.g., those on pages 66, 68 (Table 9.1), 76, and 83, on the basis of Table 6.1. For example, he equates August 6 with the nature of pure Fire, when the Sun enters the 15th degree of Leo, because August 6 is the mean between August 1 (according to Table 6.1, when the Sun enters the 10th degree of Leo) and August 11 (according to Table 6.1, when the Sun enters the 20th degree of Leo). Readers who would like to adopt Mavéric's system are advised to update this table with the aid of an ephemeris. —*Trans.*]

7

Theory of Astral Medicine in Light of the Four Humoral Temperaments

Newborns receive from their parents a spiritual and physical legacy whose indeterminate origin dates back to the distant past when their first ancestors copulated. Newborns are therefore the decided realizations of the previous influences transmitted to them by their parents at the precise moment of birth, and the astral influences recorded in their natal chart represent a fixation of the planetary influx at the moment and place of birth, which contains in a latent state the astral potentialities toward which they will gravitate over the course of their lives and to which they will succumb, but only insofar as their original atavistic nature is more or less in accord with the influences recorded in their natal chart. This explains radically why many subjects born at the same time and in the same location have drastically dissimilar destinies.

Prognostication is thus limited to determinations of the nature of the future influences revealed in the natal chart and their periods of manifestation, but such determinations cannot predict what effectual value these influences will have on the subject. The practitioner can make a rational judgment only by comparing the subject's initial nature with that of the astral influences revealed in the natal chart. From this relationship a person's destiny may be deduced, but only Mages are truly capable of making such deductions.

In the face of this uncertainty, the conscientious physician must acquire a perfect knowledge of the external character and inner nature that determine each temperament. Equipped with this knowledge, the practitioner should compare the present temperament of the subject with that indicated by their natal chart and, if they differ, calculate by means of the *primary and secondary directions* the point in time when these two temperaments will be identical. The period when the two temperaments are dissimilar generally occurs between ages 15 and 30, when the stars exert their greatest influence over the subject. Normally, the temperament is *phlegmatic* during childhood, *sanguine* during adulthood, *choleric* in middle age, and *melancholic* in old age. Childhood ranges from ages 0 to 15, adulthood from ages 15 to 30, middle age from 30 to 50, and old age from 50 to death. These figures, it must be stressed, are only approximate. If the temperament evolves in a natural way, the practitioner can predict, after an examination of the subject with respect to their age, the moment in time when their temperament will coincide with that indicated by the natal chart.

When the practitioner has determined the subject's humoral nature and evolutionary orientation, they must prescribe a vegetable diet having an elemental nature opposite that of whichever humor tends to predominate in the subject's temperament. This treatment derives from allopathic medicine and accords with the aphorism *contraria contrariis curantur,* which is to say that it restores humoral equilibrium through the ingestion of foods having an elemental nature opposite that of the dominant humor. However, unlike modern medicine, this balancing diet is preventative, and it should be prescribed only in an anodyne manner *before* the acute period breaks out.

The error of current allopathic practice, which, as we have said, does not rest on a firm foundation, is to intervene during the acute period *after* an illness has manifested. This is all the more dangerous because modern remedies are merely undeveloped or dead chemicals that are clearly dissonant with the nature of the human organism. On the contrary, the curato-preventative and balancing diet prescribed *contaria contrariis* is consonant with human nature, and its slow and evolutionary effect shields the body from disease and keeps the temperament in perfect equilibrium by vivifying the entire organism.

Persons whose temperament is sanguine will be immune from all maladies if they maintain humoral balance with a vegetable diet of a temperate nature and do not indulge in excesses of any kind. Furthermore, it is possible by means of a proper dietary regimen to restore equilibrium to each of the other temperaments. The essential remedies of Hermetic astral medicine are necessary only when humoral equilibrium has long since been broken and the body succumbs to the influence of a disease that has manifested in excess, in other words, when the disease has reached a period of crisis so acute that a preventive dietary regimen is powerless to fight against it. In this case, the practitioner must study the disease both in the subject and with the aid of the natal chart in order to determine its planetary nature. After this determination has been made, the practitioner must judiciously select an essence that has the same astral nature as the disease and administer it to the patient in a very small dosage, which, moreover, will not in any way impair the effectual value of the remedy. If necessary, the practitioner should not hesitate to mix several essences together in varying proportions. More often than not, a quintessence absorbed in an infinitesimal quantity will produce salutary effects.

In the administration of these essences, the practitioner must use diverse vehicles. For hot essences, use old sweet wines from Spain or the southern Mediterranean. For temperate essences, all young white wines are serviceable. Distilled thunderstorm water serves as an excellent vehicle for most essences. Water saturated with carbonic acid, seltzer water, sparkling water, and Vals water are also effective. A mixture of old *aqua vitae* with old wine or spirit of rainwater is the requisite vehicle for essences designed to cure cold and wet diseases. Here practitioners must use their best judgment. Above all, they must do their best to determine the temperament of the subject and the nature of the illness by the most subtle and suitable modes of investigation. For this reason, in order to guide the conscientious practitioner in such investigations, we shall delineate all the physical and mental particulars of each temperament. Subsequently, we shall more clearly explain Hermetic medicinal doctrine and further expound upon the best ways to administer dietary regimens and remedies in different cases.

The Nature and Formation of
the Four Temperaments

Each of the four temperaments owes its particular nature to the predominance in the human organism of one of the four humoral principles. These humors are constituent liquids whose proportional equilibrium generates health. The humoral proportion of the human body is directly related to prior astral influences, which become fixed in the nature of newborns through the intermediary of their parents.

The temperament evolves with age according to astral influences and a person's diet and habits, in other words, the kind of life inherent to the social individuality of the subject. The initial constitutive principle passed on by the parents evolves in a constructive, generative, and formative manner, whereas the astral influences provoke, solicit, and modify it. The one is propulsive, the other attractive. A person's destiny is contingent on the combination of and interaction between the two.

The four principle humors of the human organism are analogous to the four creative elements. Air (hot and wet) is naturally maturing, generative, nourishing, and balancing. It generates *blood,* the vital, fertilizing, and harmonic humor. Fire (hot and dry) is violent, active, and excessive in nature. It gives rise to *yellow bile,* the irritative, oxidizing, and febrile humor. Water (cold and wet) has an unstable, passive, and reflexive nature. It generates *phlegm,* the aqueous, cold, neutral, and inert humor. Earth (cold and dry) is retentive, concentrative, coagulative, and reactive in nature. It gives rise to *black bile,* the heavy, dark, atonic, and fixative humor.

8

Physiological and Psychological Analogies of the Four Temperaments

Sanguine

Element: Air (△).

Qualities: hot and wet.

Mental characteristics: harmony, good sense, dexterity, judgment, sociability, initiative, gaiety, playfulness, tenderness, altruism, assimilation, love of pleasure, generosity.

Physical characteristics: firm flesh; robust muscles; harmonious forms; warm and supple skin; a rosy, clear, and lively complexion; a regular and normal pulse; abundant capillarity; fresh breath; often brown-haired; a natural and graceful gait; a normal, saline-neutral digestion; regular organic functions; a tendency to be overweight.

Causes of imbalance: abuses of the pleasures of the table and the flesh.

Consequences: plethora, gout, local inflammations, or anemia and its side effects.

Phlegmatic

Element: Water (▽).

Qualities: cold and wet.

Mental characteristics: passivity, indifference, unconsciousness, uncertainty, indecision, submission, laziness, softness, timidity, versatility, carelessness, instability.

Physical characteristics: flaccid flesh; soft muscles; rounded forms; cold and wet skin; a pale and pallid complexion; a weak, soft, and slow pulse; average capillarity; bad breath; often blond-haired; short in stature; a timid, awkward, or nonchalant gait; abundant saliva and urine; a slow, nauseated digestion; weak organic functions in the stomach, cerebellum, and neck.

Causes of imbalance: neglect of dietary regimen and hygiene, a cold and slow circulation, stomachal apathy.

Consequences: anemia, scrofula, and their side effects.

Choleric

Element: Fire (△).

Qualities: hot and dry.

Mental characteristics: spontaneity, violence, partiality, vanity, irritability, susceptibility, feverishness, activity, audacity, presumption, courage, temerity, passion, enthusiasm, pride, irascibility, generosity.

Physical characteristics: strong flesh; well-defined, protruding muscles; angular forms; hot and dry skin; a yellow-colored complexion; a strong, violent, and irregular pulse; average capillarity; feverish breath; often brown-haired; a fast, hectic, and uneven gait; a fast, alkaline digestion; ardent thirst; sudden and impetuous appetites.

Causes of imbalance: excessive organic oxidation, feverish vitality, violence, and anger.

Consequences: bilious and hepatic overflows and renal failure.

Melancholic

Element: Earth (▽).

Qualities: cold and dry.

Mental characteristics: melancholy, prudence, reserve, modesty, concentrated pride, parsimony, persistence, moderation, meditation, deduction, circumspection, hypochondria, asceticism, solitude.

Physical characteristics: dry flesh; anemic muscles; rough and dry skin; a gray, dull, and earthy complexion; a weak and irregular pulse;

cold feet and hands; rare capillarity; acidic breath; often a gray or imprecise hair color; a shy, reserved, and hesitant gait; a slow, acidic digestion; hardness of hearing; infrequent urination; capricious appetite; sudden distastes; whimsical and nervous movements.

Causes of imbalance: reduced circulatory and nutritive functions due to excesses of fixative, cold, and retentive principles.

Consequences: uremia, hypochondria, hysteria, and nervous disorders.*

The Nature of Abnormalities Generating from Excesses of the Four Humors

The blood in a normal proportion constitutes the most balanced temperament, but it is more assimilative than the other humors due to its attractive nature, so that excess alimentation (food and drink) gradually leads to plethora, the consequences of which are gout and apoplexy. Meats and wines can be especially harmful to sanguines. Venereal abuse can cause anemia and even make the sanguine phlegmatic. Such excesses also give rise to venereal and pectoral ailments. Local inflammations are common in sanguines when they deviate from their dietary regimen.

An excess of phlegm in the organism produces cold, watery principles that attenuate the vital heat of the body, weigh down the circulation, and invade the digestive tract. Such principles are formed by the stagnation of clusters of colorless and passive liquids, which give rise by putrefaction to scrofula. The lymphatic system is directly related to the dermoid functions, and hence the frequency of cutaneous affections in the lymphatic system. In a similar manner, stagnation can often engender scrofulous necrosis due to the interconnections between the dermoid and bone tissue. An excess of phlegm causes an abundant formation of pus, which results in scrofulous or purulent affections such as ulcers and adenopathy.

An excess of yellow bile in the body excites the vital combustion and

---

*According to the alchemist, astrologer, and physician Arnaldus de Villa Nova (1240–1311), a well-balanced temperament should have the following humoral proportions: 1. one-half less phlegm than blood; 2. one-half less yellow bile than phlegm; 3. one-half less black bile than yellow bile.

causes fever. Its igneous, violent, and febrile nature irritates the organism of the individual who lacks sufficient levels of cold and wet principles. Yellow bile resides in the liver and gallbladder; it activates digestion by dissolving fat and albuminoids. In excess, this humor may, after passing through the stomach where it has swept through the excremental and acidic residues of digestion, invade the circulation and intoxicate the whole organism. It is most often the cause of jaundice, engorgement of the liver, hepatic pains, lesions, gallstones, effusions, cirrhosis, hypertrophies, and blood poisoning. The effects of anger, which in the choleric temperament is swift and violent, can be a perpetual menace. Nor is the renal system exempt from the attacks of excess yellow bile.

Of the four humors, black bile is the least vital. Its nature is atonic, fixative, and opposed to that of the blood. It is an inert and heavy humor, a byproduct of the functional residues of the organism. When such residues are in abundance, it is a clear sign of excess black bile. In this case, the albuminoid molecule undergoes, in a reducing acid medium, a retardation in the series of fermentative divisions that produce creatine, uric bodies, and leucomaines, giving rise to arthritis. Black bile slows down the eliminative functions, and hence increases urea generation and causes uremia. Its reactive, retentive, coagulative, and crystallizing nature also slows down circulation and nutrition, fixes liquids, and creates obstructions through atrophy of the assimilative functions. The special nature of these abnormalities can result in a wide range of nervous disorders, which may be classified under the following categories:

Mental neuroses: mania, vertigo, delirium, madness, insanity, obsession, nervous aphasia, abulia, epilepsy, catalepsy.

Emotional neuroses: fatigue, depression, hypochondria, nostalgia, despondency, insatiable desires, bipolar disorder, misanthropy, suicidal thoughts.

Sensory neuroses: ocular neuroses such as amaurosis, diplopia, hemianopsia, amblyopia, nyctalopia, visions, hallucinations, and hysteria; aural neuroses such as auditory hallucinations, tinnitus, and intermittent or permanent sensorineural hearing loss or nervous deafness; olfactory and gustatory neuroses such as phantom taste perception and phantosmia.

The "nervous" or melancholic humor, black bile, is therefore the origin of the vast majority of nervous disorders and diseases.

The Four Mixed Temperaments

Very few individuals belong to one of the four temperaments in an absolutely pure state. Most organisms have extremely variable humoral proportions, which is why it is necessary to examine the mixed temperaments, whose dual elemental natures are dominated by whichever quality they have in common:

1. The *choleric/sanguine temperament* (Fire/Air) is dominated by the quality of hotness in the yellow bile and blood. The result is a frequent need for subjects to seek out a brisk air or draft in order to cool down. Apoplexy threatens them after every meal.

2. The *sanguine/phlegmatic temperament* (Air/Water) is dominated by the quality of wetness in the blood and phlegm. The predominance of wetness results in excess sweating, salivation, and urination as well as wet mucous membranes and clammy skin. The subject often suffers from aquaphobia or ombrophobia.

3. The *phlegmatic/melancholic temperament* (Water/Earth) is dominated by the quality of coldness in the phlegm and black bile. Subjects are constantly cold and frequently suffer from chills. They love hot climates and loathe the winter, goosebumps, and shivering.

4. The *melancholic/choleric temperament* (Earth/Fire) is dominated by the quality of dryness in the black bile and yellow bile. Subjects often suffer from ardent thirst, dry skin, noisy and painful joints, dry mucous membranes, absence of synovium, and muscular rigidity. They love water and hydrotherapy.

The intrinsic character of each of the mixed temperaments originates exclusively from an excess in the body of one of the four elemental qualities: hot, wet, cold, or dry. Be that as it may, subjects who fall into one of these categories are not immune from diseases arising from an excess of either of the two humors that determine their mixed temperament. Thus, the patient who has a mixed temperament comprised of two joint elements may be affected by any disease corresponding to these elements, but these diseases will always be dominated by the elemental quality common to the two constitutive humors, a quality whose influence may be determined on the basis of the particular effects described above.

The Origins of Nervous Disorders

The ancients did not speak of the "nervous temperament" because this category did not exist in antiquity. But any individual is likely to experience nervous disorders as a result of a humoral imbalance. The human nervous system emits a luminous radiation that is capable of being captured by the sensitive plate of a camera or seen even more clearly by somnambulistic mediums. This radiation is nothing other than the vital, subtle, and magnetic fluid known as the *nervous influx*. The vital fluid is in direct vibratory relation with the Universal Spirit, which is itself the vital principle of the cosmos.

The Universal Spirit acts exclusively in a *hot* and *wet* environment. This environment, in which the vivifying virtue of the Universal Spirit is exalted, is maturing, generative, and digestive in nature. On the contrary, the atonic principles of the *cold* and the *dry* restrict the Universal Spirit and neutralize it, without, however, destroying it. When the human temperament is cold and dry in nature, the vital fluid or nervous influx can no longer be nourished by the Universal Spirit, since it is neutralized, and their reciprocal vibration can no longer occur except imperfectly. Hence, nervous disorders are born in melancholic temperaments whose cold and dry nature is unfavorable to reception of the *Spiritus Mundi*.

These disturbances, however, can also be born in phlegmatic temperaments through an excess of the *cold* and in choleric temperaments through an excess of the *dry*, whereas they never affect sanguine temperaments, whose hot and wet nature is conducive to the ingress of the Universal Spirit, which affords sufficient proof of this vibratory process. We have already listed the types of nervous disorders born of the melancholic temperament. The following nervous maladies are caused by excesses of phlegm or yellow bile in the human body.

Nervous Disorders Born of an Excess of Phlegm

Phlegm has a special action on the sensory nerves and is intimately tied to the digestive and circulatory functions. The phlegmatic vessels flow into the serous and passive tissues and sometimes inundate them with cold liquids. If these cold liquids should accumulate and form into centers of atonic principles and refrigerants, they will slowly flow into the organism and cause profound disturbances. Phlegm influences the stomach, the ganglionic nervous system, the dermoid system, blood circulation, and the sensory nerves. An excess of phlegm causes the following nervous disorders:

Alimentary neuroses: dyspepsia, cyclic vomiting syndrome, nervous urination and defecation, hyperesthesia, anesthesia, bladder paralysis.

Respiratory neuroses: convulsive coughs, nervous hiccups, pertussis or whooping cough.

Circulatory neuroses: migraines, neuralgia, cephalalgia, local paralysis, tremors, paralysis of the neck, pectorals, or abdominal and lumbar regions.

Generative neuroses: impotence, nymphomania, hysteria.

Perspiratory neuroses: diaphoresis or cold sweats, hyperhidrosis or nervous sweats, goosebumps, convulsive chills, pruritus.

Nervous Disorders Born of an Excess of Yellow Bile

The stomach, liver, intestines, and heart, as well as the nerve regions surrounding these organs, all fall under the direct influence of yellow bile. This humor also affects the vasomotor nerves. Nor are the pancreas, kidneys, and bladder exempt from the attacks of excess yellow bile. An excess of yellow bile can cause the following nervous disorders:

Alimentary neuroses: loss of appetite, pica or depraved appetite, bulimia, nervous hunger, gastralgia.

Circulatory neuroses: nervous heart palpitations, syncope, vertigo.

Motor neuroses (caused by continued high febrility): neuralgia, sciatica, tetanus, chorea, cramps, paresthesia, contractures, hemiplegia, paraplegia, crossed paralysis.

Generative neuroses: satyriasis, priapism.

Humoral and Organic Corruptions

The carnivorous diet is the principal cause of all humoral and organic corruptions. In fact, the vast majority of infectious diseases can be traced to such a diet. There are, however, other causes for certain epidemics and contagions. The lack of personal or collective hygiene, for example, is one of these causes, and not the least of them. Venereal diseases, moreover, have their origin in uncleanliness in sexual intercourse.

But all these diseases and all these corruptions are rooted in higher, more distant and ephemeral causes, for, in reality, all these abnormalities spring from dissonances between astral influences and the initial nature of individuals. Cures for the most serious infectious diseases cannot be easily obtained via vegetable quintessences. In such cases it is necessary to resort to mineral quintessences, to which we plan to devote a future study.[1]

9

The Hermetic Diet

The way forward, then, is to maintain humoral balance through an appropriate vegetable diet. This is not only the surest and safest treatment, but one that lies within everyone's reach.

It is possible, however, that through negligence humoral imbalance can become so great that an appropriate dietary regimen alone is powerless to restore equilibrium. In this case, it is necessary to resort to the plant preparations provided in this work and apply them according to the aphorism of sympathy, because the virtues of these medicines are more exalted and matured than those of unprepared plants and, as a result, will have more powerful and expeditious effects. Allopathic treatments utilizing such ingredients can also rapidly restore imbalanced humors to their normal and natural proportions.*

Once the temperament is well-balanced and sanguine in nature, the single best regimen one can follow is a moderate vegetable diet that varies slightly according to the seasons and consists of foods and drinks having the elemental nature opposite that of the current season. This is the path to true health.

---

*It is interesting to note that natives of a particular region will always find the foods and drinks best suited to their nature *in their country of origin*. However, subjects suffering a humoral imbalance may speed up the recovery process by living, ideally, in a country whose climate is of a nature opposite that of the predominant temperament. The following list provides orientations for countries whose climates are of a nature opposite that of each temperament: 1. *predominance of blood:* western countries, which are cold and dry; 2. *predominance of phlegm:* southern countries, which are hot and dry; 3. *predominance of yellow bile:* northern countries, which are cold and wet; 4. *predominance of black bile:* eastern countries, which are hot and wet.

Hermetic Application of the Medicinal Doctrine
Contraria contrariis curantur

The aphorism of antipathy directs one to cure the illness by its opposite, but this medicinal treatment, as we have said, is only preventive: its purpose is to maintain humoral balance or to restore the humors to their natural proportions. Applied judiciously, this treatment keeps the temperament in perfect balance and prevents the onset of illness. The ideal temperament is sanguine, and the treatment prescribed must always aim to bring the subject back to this ideal temperament.

The best way to keep the body in perfect health is to apply this aphorism by means of a diet consisting of qualities that are opposite those of the temperament's dominant humor. The sanguine temperament, which is normative, can be maintained by a vegetable diet that is neither too wet nor too hot, nor too salty. It is necessary, however, that the sanguine remain sober. The choleric temperament should be tempered by a diet that is cold and wet in nature and composed of plants that are slightly acidic. The phlegmatic temperament should be tempered by a diet that is hot and dry in nature and composed of aromatic and salty plants. Finally, the melancholic temperament should be tempered by a diet that is hot and wet in nature and composed of refreshing, fortifying, and alkaline or sugary plants.

What follows is an updated version of our earlier classification of the elemental natures of the principal comestible plants.[1] The reader will notice that there is no category for "cold and dry foods." This is not only because they are anti-vital, but because the normative sanguine temperament does not require a contrary diet.

Very Hot and Dry Foods and Herbs

Dried walnuts, dried hazelnuts, dried almonds, cocoa, chocolate, sugar, mustard, peppers, chili peppers, chili powder, nutmeg, clove, gingerbread.

Hot and Dry Foods

All cereals and dry, floury vegetables; potato starch; corn starch and corn flour; maize; chestnuts; millet; rice; buckwheat; barley; rye; wheat; oats; malted oats; peas; dried kidney beans; dried fava beans; lentils;

cassava; all pastas: macaroni, noodles, semolina, vermicelli; tapioca; dried juliennes; onions, dried onions; garlic.

Hot and Wet Foods

Dried fruits such as dried apricots and dried figs; dates; fruit jellies, jams, marmalades; French fries; roasted chestnuts; honey; fresh walnuts; prunes, raisins; brown bread, white bread.

Temperate and Wet Vegetables

Artichoke, carrot, celery, chervil, ceps, mushrooms, sauerkraut, Brussels sprouts, cauliflower, kale, spinach, flageolets, green fava beans, fresh green beans, fresh onions, sorrel, leeks, peas, potatoes, salsify, truffles.

Temperate and Wet Fruits

Apricots; sweet almonds; all common fruits: pineapples, bananas, nectarines, cherries, figs, lemons, pomegranates, strawberries, raspberries, gooseberries, tangerines, water chestnuts, oranges, peaches, apples, pears, plums, grapes.

Cold and Wet Vegetables

Domestic salads and cucurbits, lettuce, romaine, melon, asparagus, purslane, endive, chicory, eggplant, watercress, radishes, escarole, tomatoes, beetroot, cooked green beans, and especially cucumber.

Temperate and Wet
Alcoholic Beverages

Beer, pale ale, porter, cider.

Hot and Wet
Alcoholic Beverages and Liquors

Ordinary wines, natural rum, brandy, calvados.

Vegetable Drinks

In the preventative diet, beverages should occupy as important a place as solid foods because their wet nature is marvelously suited to the dry nature of certain temperaments. The following list itemizes the types of drinks apposite to each temperament:

Sanguine: temperate drinks such as young and light wines; vegetable broths and broths made from temperate fruits that are not excessively wet like garlic, chervil, green beans, fresh onions, peas, and especially apricots, dates, and dried figs, in addition to honey, prunes, and raisins. The sanguine's dietary regimen should be varied but simple.

Phlegmatic: hot and dry drinks such as old wines or Spanish wines; hot and dry vegetable broths made from oats, rye, wheat, corn, chestnuts, rice, buckwheat, barley, peas, kidney beans, lentils, and dried fava beans; Italian pasta soups; and, on occasion, old alcoholic drinks after meals.

Choleric: cold and wet drinks such as naturally acidic mineral waters; broths made from common salads such as asparagus, endive, and watercress, as well as melon, squash, pumpkin, and cucumber; acidic fruit juices such as lemon, orange, gooseberry, raspberry, and cherry.

Melancholic: hot and wet drinks such as ripe wines and generous wines; alkaline mineral waters; vegetable broths made from hot or temperate and wet plants such as artichoke, carrot, celery, chervil, sauerkraut, kale, Brussels sprouts, cauliflower, spinach, green fava beans, fresh green beans, fresh onions, leeks, salsify, and especially waters infused with hot and wet fruits such as dried figs, raisins, and prunes; in addition to fruit juices made from apricots, cherries, figs, strawberries, raspberries, pomegranates, peaches, apples, pears, plums, and fresh grapes. All acidic plants are to be avoided.*

In addition to considerations of the elemental qualities in prescriptions of preventative diets, the judicious practitioner must also take into account the secondary substances in foods revealed by chemical analyses, a subject on which numerous books have been published. Hydrocarbon, for example, which is the reconstitutive principle par excellence, is particularly well suited to phlegmatics and melancholics. Albumin, which is much less necessary to the organism than previously thought, is detrimental to phlegmatics. Acids are generally harmful to the stomach, but while cholerics can usefully absorb anodyne acids, they are detrimental to melancholics.

---

*The cabbage family in particular should be avoided if the subject is arthritic or herpetic.

Fats are heavy, and only certain cholerics can tolerate them, but sugar can be dangerous for cholerics, who exhibit a tendency toward diabetes. Stimulant drinks such as coffee, tea, and liquors can be dangerous and should be consumed only when the subject requires a temporary surplus of energy. Strictly speaking, only the phlegmatic should consume these drinks, and only in moderation. One should drink very little while eating, but one can drink a lot and without inconvenience two hours after a meal, and this applies especially to hot and dry temperaments.

The Seasonal Diet

Each of the four seasons, as we have already mentioned, has its own elemental nature. Spring is analogous to Air (wet and hot), summer to Fire (hot and dry), autumn to Earth (dry and cold), and winter to Water (cold and wet). The maximum purity of each elemental nature falls not at the beginning of the season but at its midpoint. For example, spring begins on March 20, but is not analogous to pure Air until May 5, when the Sun is in the 15th degree of Taurus (see Table 9.1 on page 68).

Whichever diet one follows, the regimen should be modified in such a manner that it gradually acquires the elemental nature opposite that of the current season until it reaches its midpoint (or pure elemental nature), after which the contrary nature of the diet should gradually decrease until the end of the season, becoming normative once more in order to adapt to the coming season.

We can reduce all this to a very simple formula: *Exalt the diet during the season whose elemental nature is analogous to that of the temperament. Attenuate the diet during the season whose elemental nature is opposed to that of the temperament.*

The Ideal Dietary Regimen

We have said that the disciple of Hermes must practice purification on the spiritual, psychical, and physical planes simultaneously. Physical purification requires a rigorous vegetarian diet. Those who advocate eating the flesh of animals often cite the fact that the human jaw is equipped with canines. But one need only draw attention to the fact that apes and monkeys, whose canines are much more developed than human canines, are exclusively frugivorous. Furthermore, the appendix with which we are equipped is found solely in vegetarian animals.

Proponents of a carnivorous diet will still cite examples of carnivorous animals such as the spider, and so on. But such examples prove only one thing, namely that these animals are made to feed on the flesh of other animals. As for human beings, it is an indisputable fact that they have *vegetarian origins*. Whoever desires to rise above the common masses should not seek to imitate animals, in which the instinct reigns supreme. Quite the contrary, one must set about vitiating that impure and gross instinct which annihilates the mental faculties in favor of a base and ignoble egoism that is firmly rooted in the earth. Universal matter continually evolves toward perfection, the pure emerges from the impure via putrefaction, which kills the body and frees the spirit. Life is born of feculent chaos, and the soul rises heavenward from vile and inert matter. Whoever wishes to acquire some notion of the higher worlds must first free themselves from the bonds of material instinct in order the better to contemplate divine works.

The consumption of animal foods is, as we have already stated, the cause of all organic corruptions. It incites humans toward their instinctive inclinations. It is the origin of all ugliness and deformity in humankind.* Cruelty, barbarity, lust, and crime are all byproducts of carnivorism. The TRUE, the GOOD, and the BEAUTIFUL sprout and stem from vegetarianism.

Tripartite individual purification is quintessential to Hermetic evolution, which confers on the disciple the numinous notions of first and second causes and their analogical effects on all universal planes.

Hermetic Application of the Medicinal Doctrine
Similia similibus curantur

The aphorism of sympathy directs one to cure the illness by its like. Here is one of the greatest mysteries of nature, and yet it is one of its most

---

*The ingestion of cheeses, for example, is the cause of most intestinal infections.

natural laws. To apply this medicinal doctrine judiciously the practitioner need only know the correspondences and analogies that link the higher worlds to the various subjects of creation. *As below, so above, and as above, so below. With this knowledge alone you may work miracles.*[2]

All human afflictions originate from past and present astral influences. Every illness is the result of humoral imbalance. Every humoral imbalance has an elemental nature, and every elemental nature has its analogies in the planetary worlds and in the three kingdoms of nature. All humoral corruptions result from dissonances between the initial nature of newborns and the nature of their planetary influences. Therefore, when humoral equilibrium is broken or altered to such an extent that an elemental dietary regimen cannot restore or purify it, it is necessary to determine the astral nature of the illness and to ascertain its analogies in the terrestrial world.

The practitioner must then select plants whose planetary nature is analogous to that of the illness,* harvest them at the appropriate time, extract from them an admirable quintessence by means of the spagyric art, and administer it to the patient under favorable celestial conditions and in the requisite vehicle. This formula results in rapid and lasting cures, because the laws of universal harmony are so designed that the mixed bodies of the microcosm assimilate and attenuate the analogous vibrations of the macrocosm, and their mutual influence is neutralized by the equilibrating law of complementarity.

TABLE 9.1.
THE PURE ELEMENTAL NATURES OF THE SEASONS

Season	Pure Element	Date	Position of Sun
Spring	Pure Air (△)	May 5	☉ in 15° ♉
Summer	Pure Fire (△)	August 6	☉ in 15° ♌
Autmn	Pure Earth (▽)	November 6	☉ in 15° ♏
Winter	Pure Water (▽)	February 5	☉ in 15° ♒

---

*Consult the astral correspondences of plants in chapter 6.

10

Planetary Natures and Their Analogies on the Physical and Mental Planes

The Sun (☉)

The Sun is the active, dynamic, and caloric center. It is the origin of the simultaneous rectilinear and circular double motion of repulsion and attraction.

Planetary radiation: electropositive radiation of a violent, excessive, irritative, and masculine nature.

Nature of functions: violence, excitement, diffusion, volatilization, fertilization, animation, vivification, excitement, exaltation.

Elemental analogy: Fire (more hot than dry).

Temperament: choleric (hot).

Mental analogies: pride, expansion, generosity, nobility, violence, authority, enthusiasm, ambition, magnanimity, domination.

Physical analogies: heart, arteries, great sympathetic nervous system, vasomotor nerves, dextrality, sense of sight, general regulation of organic functions.

The Moon (☾)

The Moon is the passive center of reflection and transmission, the receptor and moderator of the solar influx.

Planetary radiation: magneto-negative radiation of an attenuating, passive, neutral, and feminine nature.

Nature of functions: attenuation, moderation, humidification, formation, gestation, transmission, reflection.

Elemental analogy: Water (more cold than wet).

Temperament: phlegmatic (cold).

Mental analogies: passivity, femininity, submission, inconstancy, docility, versatility, gentleness, indifference, imagination, instability, carelessness.

Physical analogies: lymphatic, digestive, and generative systems, lymphatic vein, cerebellum, quadri-luminal tubercles, serous and passive tissues, stomach, nipples, throat, intestine, womb, bladder, sinistrality, sense of taste.

Saturn (♄)

Saturn is the fixative, atonic, and structural principle.

Planetary radiation: magneto-positive radiation of a slow, concentrative, deep, and durable nature.

Nature of functions: retention, reaction, concentration, coagulation, crystallization, agglomeration, rigidity, fixation.

Elemental analogy: Earth (more cold than dry).

Temperament: melancholic (cold).

Mental analogies: concentration, moderation, reserve, deduction, caution, personal egoism, taciturnity, hypochondria, envy, parsimony, perseverance.

Physical analogies: bone structure, cartilage, vertebrae, joints, spleen, bladder, legs, feet, teeth, heavy humors, black bile, inanition, chronic diseases, sense of gravity.

Jupiter (♃)

Jupiter is the assimilative, compensatory, and balancing principle.

Planetary radiation: electropositive radiation of a tempering, generative, evolutive, and maturing nature.

Nature of functions: moderation, regularization, maturation, evolution, assimilation, growth, generation.

Elemental analogy: Air (more hot than wet).

Temperament: sanguine (balanced, or "hot sanguine").

Mental analogies: judgment, dignity, loyalty, ambition, pride, benevolence, love of honor and fortune, moral sense.

Physical analogies: blood, arterial circulation, regulation of assimilative functions (myotrophy, respiration, digestion), pulmonary parenchyma, pectoralis major and minor, portal vein, seminal secretion, diaphragm, intercostal muscles, sense of balance.

Mars (♂)

Mars is the active principle of selfishness.

Planetary radiation: electropositive radiation of an irritative, violent, virile, febrile, and intermittent nature.

Nature of functions: action, activity, erethism, desiccation, penetration.

Elemental analogy: Fire (more dry than hot).

Temperament: choleric (dry).

Mental analogies: violence, irascibility, tyranny, passion, cruelty, courage, temerity, presumption, audacity, jealousy, vanity, contradiction, susceptibility.

Physical analogies: muscular and virile system, liver, yellow bile, gall, penis, kidneys, adrenal capsules, lower jaw, fourth ventricle, anus, sense of touch.

Venus (♀)

Venus is the principle of harmony and attraction.

Planetary radiation: magneto-negative radiation of an attractive, harmonic, attenuating, homogeneous, and sweet nature.

Nature of functions: attenuation, moderation, generation, love, attraction.

Elemental analogy: Air (more wet than hot).

Temperament: sanguine/phlegmatic (or "cold sanguine").

Mental analogies: love, sensuality, altruism, voluptuousness, sociability, susceptibility, sensitivity, charm, joy, gaiety, intuition, compassion, charity, indulgence, artistic sense.

Physical analogies: feminine principle of sensuality and generation, inner sex, uterine and vaginal fluids, ovaries, uterus, kidneys, testicles, breasts, mammary glands, thyroid gland, pharynx, throat, complexion, sense of smell.

Mercury (☿)

Mercury is the principle of sensation, perception, and motion.

Planetary radiation: electromagnetic radiation of a subtle, variable, penetrating, mobile, and spiritual nature.

Nature of functions: rarefaction, acceleration, transmission, perception, assimilation, spiritualization.

Elemental analogy: Earth (more dry than cold).

Temperament: melancholic (dry).

Mental analogies: subtlety, ingenuity, initiative, adaptation, deduction, intuition, promptness, rationality, diplomacy, cleverness.

Physical analogies: central nervous system, spinal cord, solar plexus, sensory and motor nerves, facial nerves, larynx, pectoralis major and minor, intestinal innervation, encephalon, gallbladder, sense of hearing.

Uranus (♅)

Uranus is the principle of disintegration and discarnation.

Planetary radiation: electromagnetic radiation of a dissonant, intermittent, and abnormal nature.

Elemental nature: negatively cold and dry.

Physical analogy: the nervous influx.

Neptune (♆)

Neptune is the passive principle of involution and retrogression.

Planetary radiation: magneto-negative radiation of a subtle, immutable, foreign, disturbing, absorbent, and fatal nature.

Elemental nature: negatively temperate and wet.

Physical analogy: the medianimic fluid.

The two planets Uranus and Neptune are dissonant on the physical plane but harmonic on the spiritual plane.

The Influence of the Planets
on the Organic Functions
of the Human Body

The Sun is vital, active, and dynamic. It is the origin of double motion, which is analogous to the systole and diastole of the cardiac cycle. Its vital principle spreads throughout the entire body via the heart, the vasomotor nerves, and the great sympathetic nervous system.

The Moon is the passive and feminine receptor of the solar influx, which it reflects and transmits in a temperate manner. It presides over the female generative organs, which are likewise passive and receptive in nature, and governs the functions of nutrition by its action on the stomach and intestinal mucous membranes. The Moon is fertilized by the Sun, whose seed it nourishes and forms by gestation in the salty mother liquor.

Saturn coagulates the dissolved salt to form bones. It solidifies the soft tissues, fixes the passive liquids, and determines their specifications. It tempers the violent and feverish natures of the Sun and Mars and retains the mobile natures of the Moon and Mercury with its cold, dry, and retentive qualities. Saturn gives body to the tissues, fibers, nerves, and ligaments. It moderates the warm and alkaline nature of the yellow bile with its cold acidity. It nourishes and consolidates the bone structure.

Jupiter is the compensator of humoral balance. It presides over the oxygenation and circulation of the blood. It nourishes the muscles and tones the tissues. Its maturing and generous nature regulates the functions of assimilation and attenuates dissonances caused by other planets.

The active and hot nature of Mars animates the cold and humid influence of the Moon and the atonic influence of Saturn. It activates and strengthens the muscles and stimulates digestion by its action on the yellow bile. Its virile nature arouses sexual desire, which makes it the primary cause of generation. It stimulates the eliminative functions by its action on the kidneys and compensates for the passive feminine natures of the Moon and Venus.

Venus harmonizes the general functions of the body and especially the organs of generation. It partly alleviates the feverish and violent influences of the Sun and Mars and combats the hypochondria of

Saturn. It incites love and generation through the attractive influence it spreads over all creatures. It is she who exalts feminine sensuality.

Mercury governs the transmitting, perceptor, and motor organs. It transforms the will from potentiality into actuality and informs the brain of external sensations. It controls and coordinates the motor and sensory nervous system with the spinal cord and the brain. It is the principle of central innervation.

A comprehensive knowledge of these analogies is indispensable to an accurate analysis of the patient's natal chart.[1]

Fundamental Rules for Investigating Maladies in the Natal Chart

The measure and nature of the aspects and their orbs relative to planetary radiation are given in our *Essai synthétique*.[2] The aspects of the planets must be carefully determined and studied according to the following guidelines, because they are, more or less, the principal causes of harmony and disharmony in the natal chart:

1. The vibration of consonant aspects conjoins and unites the shared elemental qualities of the aspected planets in a harmonic manner and tempers the elemental qualities of opposed natures.
2. The vibration of dissonant aspects partially neutralizes the shared elemental qualities of the aspected planets while exalting the violently clashing elemental qualities of opposed natures.
3. The variable aspects act like the conjunction, but with less power.

Determinations of illnesses are based on the dissonant aspects of the vital significators. Each planet has an intimate nature and an elemental nature, both of which act upon all levels of creation. Modifications in the intimate natures of the planets derive from their mutual aspects and their respective positions in the signs and houses, but variations brought about in their elemental natures derive primarily from their aspects to the Sun and the Moon, as we shall later demonstrate. The vital significators are the Sun, the Moon, planets in the hylegiacal places, and especially Jupiter and Venus. The hylegiacal places are those in which the planetary influx has the most vital action on the subject at the moment of birth, whereas the anaretic places are those in which the planetary influx is abnormal or neutral.

The Vital Cycle (Fig. 11.5 on page 90) provides the values of vitality for the four angles and the twelve houses in the natal chart. This cycle only provides the coefficients of vitality for the places or houses, but certain places or houses may have additional beneficent or maleficent influences on a person's life. Thus, houses I, X, XI, IX, and VII are the most favorable to the vitality, whereas houses VIII, VI, and XII are always harmful to the life and vitality of the subject. Planets positioned in the latter three houses, and especially Saturn and Mars, are particularly unfavorable to the vitality, and all the more so if they negatively aspect one or more of the vital significators or hylegs.

The elements of the natal chart relate, in a general way, to each humoral nature: *blood* corresponds to Jupiter, Venus, Air signs, and the Ascendant (Asc); *yellow bile* to the Sun, Mars, Fire signs, and Midheaven (MC); *phlegm* to the Moon, Venus, Water signs, and the Nadir (IC); and *black bile* to Saturn, Mercury, Earth signs, and the Descendant (Dsc).

Nervous disorders derive from the maleficent aspects that Mercury receives from Saturn and Uranus in the Earth signs and near the Descendant. Cerebral disturbances derive from the maleficent aspects that Mercury receives from Neptune in the proximities of the four angles and especially in whichever zodiacal sign happens to govern the subject's head.

The sixth house, the planets occupying it, and its ruling planet are the most likely indicators of illness in the natal chart, and hence these are the best places to look for diseases. By analogy the twelfth house has a similarly maleficent character. The practitioner should note their relationships to the hylegs and to any planets situated in the first house.*

Orientation of the Natal Chart

Any astrologer who has worked with a number of charts will know that the traditional correspondence of the zodiacal sign Aries with the

---

*Any physician who would be unscrupulous enough to treat a patient according to a natal chart drafted other than by precise astronomical calculations would assume a heavy responsibility indeed.

human head is false nine times out of ten. However, no author has shed any light on this obscure point, and what we have previously written on the matter is inconclusive.

The problem is all the more difficult to solve because the fundamental bases of astrology, as the Arabs and their successors have transmitted them, are obviously false, at least in part. Thus, the traditional elemental succession of the signs is not only impossible but even contrary to universal laws. No law of nature is capable of manifestation except in a natural and harmonic manner, and this is why there is never a solution of continuity in the work of creation.

According to tradition, the zodiacal signs succeed each other in the following elemental order: Fire → Earth → Air → Water → Fire, etc. Now, if Fire (hot and dry) is linked to Earth (cold and dry) by the common quality of dryness, then this leaves no qualitative connection or transition between Earth (cold and dry) and Air (hot and wet). Likewise, if Air (hot and wet) is linked to Water (cold and wet) by the common quality of wetness, then this leaves no qualitative connection between Water (cold and wet) and Fire (hot and dry). As a result, there are two solutions of continuity in the traditional elemental succession of the signs. These two solutions of continuity are absolutely contrary to universal laws, and they occur three times each within the zodiacal circle. In order for the succession of signs to flow naturally, the elemental order must proceed as follows: Air → Fire → Earth → Water → Air, etc., according to the order of the four seasons. We hope to study this matter in greater detail in a separate work.

Additional proof of corruption in the transmitted tradition lies in the arbitrary manner in which the signs are attributed to planets as domiciles. Thus, to cite just one example, astrological tradition correctly places the Sun in its domicile in the 15th degree of Leo because the heat wave occurs during this time of the year (August 6), which corresponds to the nature of pure Fire. But tradition places the Moon in the domicile of Cancer and thereby removes it from its true cold and wet nature: the Sun transits Cancer during the month of July, which is hot and dry. The true domicile of the Moon is in the 15th degree of Aquarius (February 5), which is the coldest and wettest time of the year. Moreover, the Moon, which is the complementary principle of the Sun, now sits in its domicile (☾ in 15° ♒) in diametrical opposition to the Sun in its domicile (☉ in 15° ♌), and this opposition perfectly reflects their opposing natures, whose equilibrium is the cause of generation. Many other aspects of traditional astrology require similar revision, but this is a task to which we shall devote ourself in the future.[3]

Nevertheless, we have developed a logical and rational method of orienting the natal chart by first determining the zodiacal sign that corresponds to the subject's head. The *Aries–Head* correspondence serves as the starting point, but this, like any synthesis, must be developed according to the laws of the Binary, Ternary, and Quaternary.

The Binary finds its application in opposition. Opposed elements are complementary, and their equilibrium is born of their opposition, from which a mixed or neutral nature is born. Thus, each astrological house is analogous to whichever house lies opposite to it. For example, the House of Self, which is the house of individuality (House I: *Vita/* Life), represents the Unity and finds its complement in its opposite, the House of Partnerships, which is the house of duality (House VII: *Uxor/* Spouse), and this constitutes the Binary. The *Aries–Head* correspondence constitutes the Unity. The *Aries–Libra–Head* correspondence constitutes the Binary.

The Ternary is the realization of the Unity on the three universal planes by the mystery of the Divine Trinity. The laws of the Ternary and Quaternary find their application in the four elemental triplicities of the zodiacal signs Fire, Water, Air, and Earth, which proceed from the Quaternary. These laws are reproduced analogically in the division of the twelve solar houses into four trilogies, for which the four angles of the natal chart serve as the bases (see Table 10.1 on page 79). The analogical laws of the Ternary and Quaternary apply quite naturally to the four elemental triplicities of the zodiac, of which the triplicity of Fire is the first and most powerful. Their applications are as follows: the *Aries–Leo–Sagittarius–Head* correspondence constitutes the Ternary; the *Aries–Four Angles–Head* correspondence constitutes the Quaternary.

Each of the three Fire signs may therefore serve as the sign corresponding to the human head in the natal chart, and by the analogical principle of opposition each Air sign can likewise serve as the sign corresponding to the human head, since the Air signs lie opposite the Fire signs. Each of the four angles may also indicate the place occupied by the head sign. In short, *the sign corresponding to the human head in the natal chart will be either a Fire sign or an Air sign, and this sign will be positioned on or very near to one of the four astrological angles.*

To identify which of the Fire or Air signs represents the head sign by its proximity to one of the four angles, first determine the position of the Sun, which signifies the place of the heart *by its presence or its opposition,* then ascend from the place of the heart (*the Sun sign or its opposing sign*) to the Fire or Air sign occupied by whichever angle represents the cusp of the house corresponding to the head. For a graphic representation, consult the dial showing the succession of the parts and organs of the human body through each of the houses, starting with the angle that occupies the head sign (Fig. 10.1).

Once you have determined the house of the head by the angle positioned in the sign that corresponds to the head, chart the rest of the parts and organs of the human body *according to the extent of the houses,* not according to the extent of the signs. The more the houses are extended, the more the human organs they represent are open to astral influences, whether they be beneficent or maleficent.

The cusp of the house corresponding to the head will therefore be one of the angles closest to one of the Fire or Air signs, depending on the Sun's position. For this to remain valid, however, it is necessary that the cusp of the angle fall within the determined sign or at least within the last degrees of the preceding sign. The Fire signs are preceded by the Water signs and the Air signs by the Earth signs. But if the cusp of the angle falls within the last three degrees of a Fire sign or Air sign, it cannot represent the sign of the head, and one will need to look elsewhere. There are instances when the position of the Sun or its opposition will correspond to the head sign, and this is why, despite everything, the practitioner must exercise a great deal of

TABLE 10.1. THE FOUR ELEMENTAL TRIPLICITIES
AND THE TWELVE HOUSES

Angles	Houses
First Trilogy: based at the Asc	I. Life in itself. V. Life in infants. IX. Life in God.
Second Trilogy: based at the Dsc	VII. Relationships of union. XI. Relationships of friendship. III. Relationships of kinship.
Third Trilogy: based at the MC	X. Social realization. II. Individual realization. VI. Auxiliary realization.
Fourth Trilogy: based at the IC	IV. Social end. VIII. Individual end. XII. Causal end.

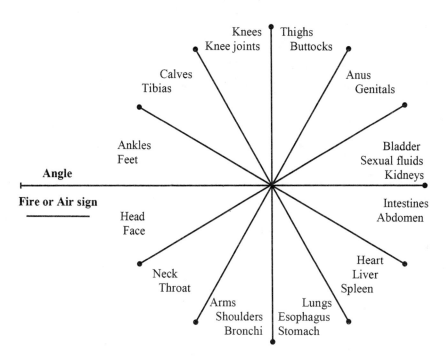

Fig. 10.1. Succession of the Parts and Organs of the Human Body
Corresponding to Each House

TABLE 10.2. CORPOREAL AND ORGANIC CORRESPONDENCES WITH THE ZODIACAL SIGNS (HOUSES THAT MAY CORRESPOND TO THE HEAD: I, VII, X, IV)

♈	♉	♊	♋	♌	♍	♎	♏	♐	♑	♒	♓
HEAD	neck	shoulders	stomach	heart	intestines	kidneys	genitals	thighs	knees	tibias	feet
		HEAD	neck	shoulders	stomach	heart	intestines	kidneys	genitals	thighs	knees
tibias	feet			HEAD	neck	shoulders	stomach	heart	intestines	kidneys	genitals
thighs	knees	tibias	feet			HEAD	neck	shoulders	stomach	heart	intestines
kidneys	genitals	thighs	knees	tibias	feet			HEAD	neck	shoulders	stomach
heart	intestines	kidneys	genitals	thighs	knees	tibias	feet			HEAD	neck
shoulders	stomach	heart	intestines	kidneys	genitals	thighs	knees	tibias	feet		

judgment in the examination of the subject's natal chart. The position of the planets in the houses can help practitioners orient the natal chart if they consider the physical correspondences of the planets and their mutual aspects.

Table 10.2 shows the various corporeal and organic successions that can occur in all possible cases. We must stress, however, that these correspondences are subordinate to the extent of the houses, because some will encompass more than one sign at a time and others will occupy only half of a sign. Furthermore, it should be obvious to readers that the parts and organs of the human body listed in the dial of correspondences (Fig. 10.1) and in the table of possible corporeal and organic successions (Table 10.2) are incomplete due to insufficient space. For this reason, we supply a more comprehensive listing of these correspondences, starting with the sign corresponding to the human head, which for practical purposes we fictitiously identify with the first house (see Table 10.3).

TABLE I0.3. THE ZODIACAL HOUSES AND THE
PARTS AND ORGANS OF THE HUMAN BODY

House I	House II	House III	House IV	House V	House VI
head	neck	arms	chest	heart	abdomen
face	inner throat	hands	lungs	arteries	intestines
(organs of	outer throat	shoulders	esophagus	diaphragm	kidneys
the head	larynx	upper lungs	stomach	back	(sometimes
and face)	pharynx	bronchi	(sometimes	flanks	the spleen)
	vocal folds	etc.	the liver and	liver	
	trachea		spleen)	spleen	
	carotids			(sometimes	
	etc.			the stomach	
				and local	
				nerves)	

House VII	House VIII	House IX	House X	House XI	House XII
bladder	genitals	hips	knees	legs	ankles
backbone	bladder	pelvis	knee joints	tibias	feet
sexual fluids	anus	femurs	(sometimes	calves	
kidneys	womb	thighs	the calves)	(sometimes	
navel	coccyx	buttocks		the ankles)	
vertebrae	groin				
uterus	pelvis				
(sometimes	hips				
the femurs)	(sometimes				
	the femurs)				

11
Mechanical Theory of Astral Vibrations

The Sun, as the active energy center of the planetary system, is the origin of positive vibrations. The Moon, as the passive reflex center of the earth system, is the origin of negative vibrations. The nature of the Sun's vibrations alters according to its position in the zodiac (the four seasons) and its position relative to the Earth (the four angles). The nature of the Moon's vibrations varies according to its position relative to the Sun and to the four angles.

The influx of these two celestial bodies mixes in varying proportions and transmutes into different vibratory modes that are more or less favorable to generation. This double influx is the principal cause of modifications in the elemental natures of the other planets, because the combined radiation of the luminaries, which alters in its nature according to the seasons and the angles, *contains this binary influence virtually within itself and transmits it to the planets.* The vital influence of the luminaries on the earthly plane is more powerful than that of all the other planets combined. The influx of the luminaries is so powerful, in fact, that it alters the initial natures of the planets, without, however, destroying them.

The entrance of the Sun into the four cardinal signs marks the beginning of each season, and each season possesses the nature of one of the four elements. But the seasons are pure in their elemental nature only at their midpoint. Thus, summer reaches the nature of pure Fire only when the Sun arrives in the 15th degree of Leo, because this is the hottest time of the year. Accordingly, winter reaches the nature of pure Water only when the Sun arrives in the 15th degree of Aquarius (directly opposite that of Leo), because this the coldest and wettest time of the year (see Fig. 9.1). To summarize, here are the annual and zodiacal correspondences for the elemental natures of the seasons:*

- **Spring** begins on March 20 when the Sun enters Aries (♈) and culminates in the nature of pure Air (wet and hot) on May 5 when the Sun reaches the 15th degree of Taurus (♉).
- **Summer** begins on June 21 upon entry of the Sun in Cancer (♋) and culminates in the nature of pure Fire (hot and dry) on August 6 when the Sun is in the 15th degree of Leo (♌).
- **Autumn** begins on September 22 when the Sun enters Libra (♎) and culminates in the nature of pure Earth (dry and cold) on November 6 when the Sun reaches the 15th degree of Scorpio (♏).
- **Winter** begins on December 21 upon entry of the Sun in Capricorn (♑) and culminates in the nature of pure Water (cold and wet) on February 5 when the Sun is in the 15th degree of Aquarius (♒).

Fig. 11.1 on page 88 charts this elemental weather pattern over the course of the year in much greater detail.

The four positions of the Sun in relation to the Horizon and the Earth Meridian are analogous to the four elements and the four seasons: *sunrise,* when the Sun is at the Asc, corresponds to the nature of Air and spring; *sunset,* when the Sun is at the Dsc, corresponds to the nature of Earth and autumn; *midday,* when the Sun is at the MC, corresponds to the nature of Fire and summer; and *midnight,* when the Sun is at the IC, corresponds to the nature of Water and winter (see Table 1.1 on page 16).

By analogy the four aspects of the Moon to the Sun or the four phases of the Moon also reflect the nature of the four elements.

---

*These dates and degrees will vary slightly in some years, but we give a fair average.

According to ancient astrologers, the conjunction (New Moon) is cold and wet, the first square (First Quarter Moon) is wet and hot, the opposition (Full Moon) is hot and dry, and the last square (Last Quarter Moon) is dry and cold. We do not share this opinion, however, for it is clear that, according to the principle of conjunctions, whichever celestial body is more powerful in quality and nature will communicate in part both its quality and its nature to the weaker celestial body. The Sun, which is the most powerful celestial body in our planetary system, communicates in part its hot and dry nature to whichever planet is in conjunction with it.

To get a good idea of the effect of the conjunctions and other aspects, we must compare these planetary natures with respect to the four seasons and the four angles. The Sun is of the nature of summer and the MC, and the Moon is of the nature of winter and the IC. These two seasons and angles are opposed to each other. The Moon will therefore be dry and hot when it is in conjunction (☌) with the Sun; in the first quarter (□) it will be hot and wet like the Asc and spring; in opposition (☍) to the Sun it will be wet and cold like the IC and winter; and in the last quarter (□) it will be cold and dry like the Dsc and autumn. Fig. 11.2 on page 89 more clearly illustrates the changes in the elemental qualities of the Moon according to its position relative to the Sun.

The luminaries thus emit a combined circular vibration of a temperate and generative nature, which balances the elemental natures of the planets. The elemental nature of this original vibration alters over the course of the year according to the influence of the four angles and the four seasons, and this results in variations in the elemental qualities of the combined vibration of the luminaries, whose immediate impression the planets receive, without, however, destroying their own natures or that of the luminaries, whose fundamental constitution is immutable.

One may therefore assume that the particular aspects of the planets to the luminaries are the primary cause of variations in their elemental natures and that this cause in itself is much more powerful than the aspects of the planets to each other or their positions relative to the four angles (at least with respect to modifications in their elemental natures). Such secondary causes may be disregarded, however, since the influx of the luminaries virtually and forcefully transmits to the planets the influences of the seasons, the angles, and their mutual aspects.

The following illustrates the effects of the luminaries on the elemental natures of the planets according to their mutual aspects:

- **Fire** in conjunction with the Sun or in opposition to the Moon intensifies the hot and dry qualities or attenuates the cold and wet qualities.
- **Water** in opposition to the Sun or in conjunction with the Moon increases the cold and wet qualities or decreases the hot and dry qualities.
- **Air** in ascending (east) quadrature to the Sun or descending (west) quadrature to the Moon intensifies the wet and hot qualities or attenuates the dry and cold qualities.
- **Earth** in descending (west) quadrature to the Sun or ascending (east) quadrature to the Moon increases the dry and cold qualities or decreases the wet and hot qualities.

Knowledge of these vibratory effects is absolutely essential in the practice of determining a person's astral temperament.

From the preceding it may rightly be deduced that since the luminaries are of opposed natures their aspects to the planets will produce opposite effects. Thus, the mutual conjunction of the luminaries partly annihilates their particular effect, while their mutual opposition increases it. This whole process becomes logical when one considers that the influx emanating from the luminaries constitutes a natural elemental medium, and one which is necessary to maintain a universal vibratory equilibrium, such that attenuation of the hot and dry qualities transmits an impression of the cold and the wet, while attenuation of the cold and wet qualities produces the opposite effect.

We must be careful, however, not to confuse the original natures of the planetary qualities with their material analogies, because they exist in a latent state of pure and embryonic spirituality and are realized on the physical plane only by transforming into constituent elements and principles. On the physical plane, the heat of the Sun is several million times stronger than that of Mars, while its elemental heat is hardly greater than that of Jupiter.

Measuring Variations in the Natures of the Planets by Their Aspects to the Luminaries

Step 1. Determine the coefficients of the elemental qualities of the natal Sun according to its position relative to the zodiac and the four angles using the special chart (Fig. 11.6 on page 91).

Step 2. Determine the coefficients of the elemental qualities of the natal Moon according to its position relative to the Sun and the four angles using Fig. 11.7 on page 92, but factor in the coefficient values of the natal Sun calculated using the Sun's special chart.

Step 3. Calculate the coefficients of the elemental qualities of each natal planet *first* according to its aspect to the Sun and *then* according to its aspect to the Moon using Figs. 11.8–12 on pages 93–95, each of which is established for an average Sun (in most charts: Hot 55, Dry 20) and an average Moon (in most charts: Wet 40, Cold 25). Do not worry about the angularity of the planets or their mutual aspects, at least as far as the coefficients of their elemental qualities are concerned.

Except for the chart of the Sun, the coefficients given in each of the planetary charts are only *averages* and must vary, for the Moon according to the elemental value of the Sun, and for the planets according to the elemental value of the luminaries. Furthermore, the average coefficients of the elemental qualities of the planets provided in Figs. 11.8–12 are relative to the aspects of the luminaries only *in isolation.* Thus, they are established either for conjunction with the Sun or for opposition to the Moon, but not for a combination of these two aspects. If, then, a planet is in conjunction with the Sun at the same time as it is in opposition to the Moon, the value of its elemental variation should be doubled, whereas it should be canceled out if the planet were in conjunction with both luminaries. It should also be noted that the coefficients are established only for aspects that are exact and pure in their elemental nature, namely conjunctions, quadratures, and oppositions, which are analogous to the four angles and the four seasons.

There are, of course, intermediate aspects which, being situated between quadrature and conjunction or opposition, participate in a single quality, namely whichever quality is common to the natures of the aforesaid aspects. Since we have already demonstrated the elemental natures of the seasons, angles, and aspects, it is unnecessary to reproduce these analogies here. It is sufficient to note that planets situated between two elemental points will be influenced by whichever quality is common to both elements. For example, Air and Fire have the common quality of hotness, Fire and Earth the common quality of dryness, Earth and Water the common quality of coldness, and Water and Air the common quality of wetness (see Figs. 11.3–4).

Calculating Variations in the Elemental Natures of the Planets

After measuring the variations in the nature of the Sun according to its position in the natal chart using the coefficient chart of the Sun (Fig. 11.6) and in the nature of the Moon according to its position relative to the Sun in the natal chart using its special chart (Fig. 11.7), pass these two measure values through the sieve of the Vital Cycle (Fig. 11.5) according to the positions of the luminaries in the twelve houses of the natal chart.

The number 50 in the Vital Cycle corresponds to the maximum vitality, which means that the newborn is entirely open to the influence of a star that is situated in this place. All other numbers are only fractions of this maximum vitality. Thus, a star situated at the number 27 would influence the newborn at only twenty-seven fiftieths of its maximum vital power. Therefore, after you have calculated the elemental coefficients of the Sun and the Moon, determine the values of their vital power in the natal chart according to their positions relative to the divisions of the Vital Cycle. This operation will further modify their elemental value, and it is this definitive value on which we must then rely when calculating the elemental value of the planets.

When this calculation has been made, pass the planetary coefficients—in the same manner as the coefficients of the luminaries—through the sieve of the Vital Cycle to obtain their exact effective values. It is important to note that the coefficients of the Vital Cycle relate to the houses and their extent, which is variable and often unequal, and should be modified proportionally according to the particular places occupied by the planets in the houses.

The above explanation of the vibratory mechanism of the stars together with the coefficient values provided in the figures below should constitute sufficiently precise bases such that the advanced student may find in them all of the necessary components for determining the values of the elemental natures of the planets according to their respective positions. With a little practice, patience, and perspicacity, the practitioner will be able to calculate these values at a fairly rapid pace.

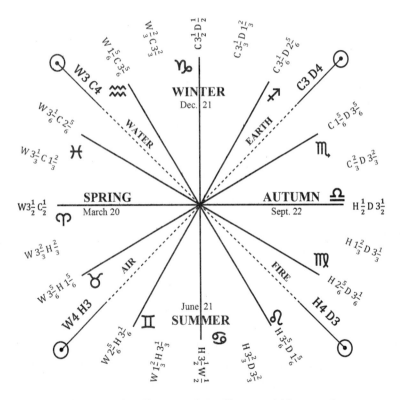

Fig. 11.1. Coefficients of the Elemental Nature of
the Sun over the Course of the Seasons

Determining a Person's Astral Temperament

After determining the qualitative coefficients of the planets using the three steps outlined above, add together all of the like qualities of each planet (luminaires included). These totals will give the precise proportion of hot, wet, cold, and dry qualities constituting the astral temperament of the subject at the moment of birth. The qualities hot and cold and the qualities dry and wet cancel each other out. As a result, one may easily determine the nature of a person's astral temperament according to the dominant proportions of two of these qualities, which together will make up one of the four elemental natures, namely Air, Fire, Earth, or Water.[1]

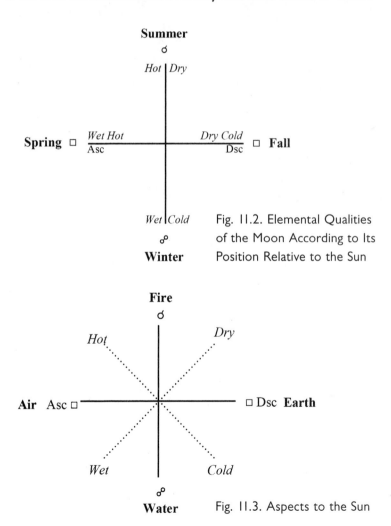

Fig. 11.2. Elemental Qualities of the Moon According to Its Position Relative to the Sun

Fig. 11.3. Aspects to the Sun

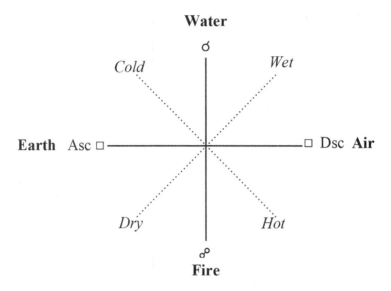

Fig. 11.4. Aspects to the Moon

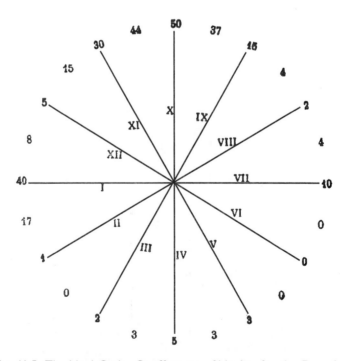

Fig. 11.5. The Vital Cycle: Coefficients of Vitality for the Four Angles
and the Twelve Houses of the Natal Chart

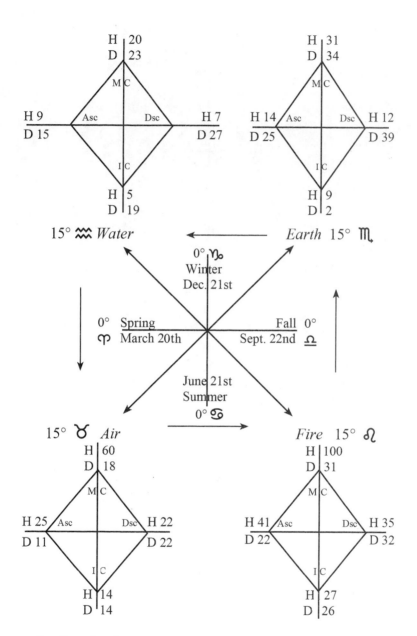

Fig. 11.6. Coefficients of the Elemental Qualities of the Sun (☉)
According to Its Position Relative to the Four Seasons and the Four Angles

*N.B.: In this and the following diagrams the letters H, W, C, and D
stand for Hot, Wet, Cold, and Dry.*

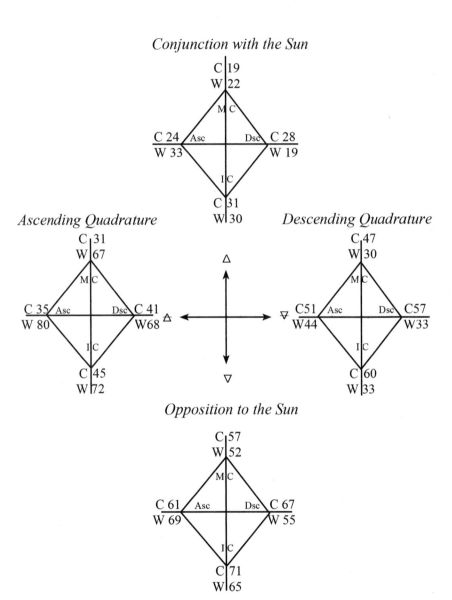

Fig. 11.7. Average Coefficients of the Elemental Qualities of the Moon (☾)
According to Its Position Relative to the Sun and the Four Angles
(Average ☉ = H 55, D 20)

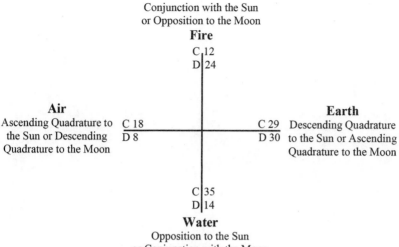

Fig. 11.8. Average Coefficients of the Elemental Qualities of Saturn (♄)
According to Its Aspects to the Sun and the Moon
(Average ☉ = H 55, D 20; Average ☾ = W 40, C 25)

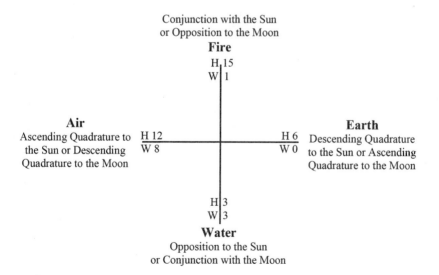

Fig. 11.9. Average Coefficients of the Elemental Qualities of Jupiter (♃)
According to Its Aspects to the Sun and the Moon
(Average ☉ = H 55, D 20; Average ☾ = W 40, C 25)

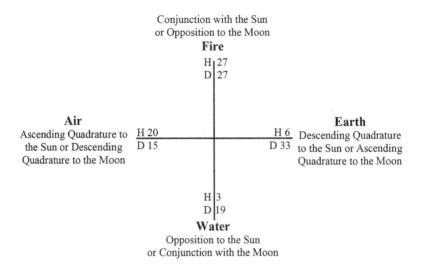

Fig. II.10. Average Coefficients of the Elemental Qualities of Mars (♂)
According to Its Aspects to the Sun and the Moon
(Average ☉ = H 55, D 20; Average ☾ = W 40, C 25)

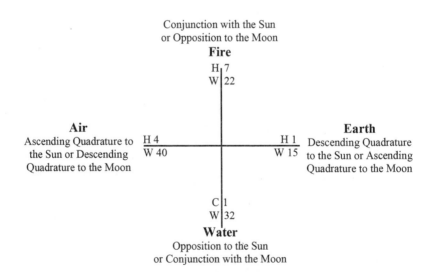

Fig. II.11. Average Coefficients of the Elemental Qualities of Venus (♀)
According to Its Aspects to the Sun and the Moon
(Average ☉ = H 55, D 20; Average ☾ = W 49, C 25)

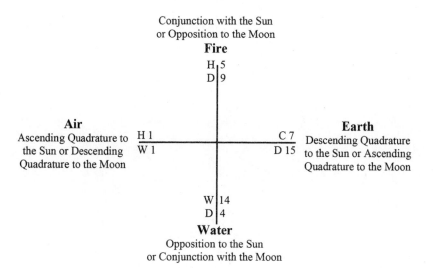

Fig. 11.12. Average Coefficients of the Elemental Qualities of Mercury (☿)
According to Its Aspects to the Sun and the Moon
(Average ☉ = H 55, D 29; Average ☽ = W 46, C 25)

PART TWO

ELEMENTARY CHEMISTRY, SPAGYRICS, AND SECRET OPERATIONS

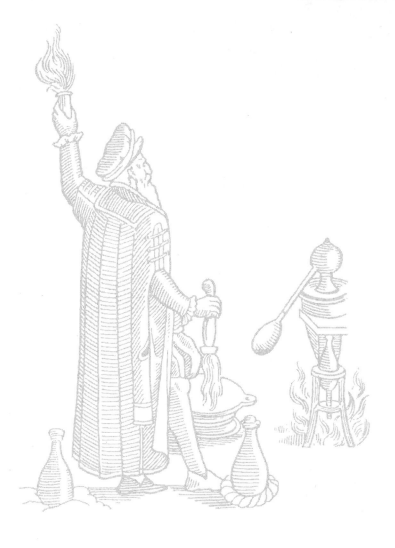

12

Principles of Premodern Chemistry for Basic Preparations of Medicinal Plants

The main agent of chemistry is fire or heat. This fire or heat can be manifested in a variety of ways. The premodern chemists distinguished seven different fires:

1. The first fire and the most innocuous is that of the *balneum vaporis* or "steam bath," which is humid in nature and is made by suspending the vessel over the steam of warm or hot water. This fire is suitable for putrefaction, fermentation, and circulation.
2. The second fire is that of the *balneum Mariae,* literally "Mary's bath,"* the water bath or bain-marie, which is made by immersing the vessel in another containing warm or hot water. This fire is hot and wet and generative in nature. It is suitable for digestion, dissolution, circulation, and slow distillation.
3. The third fire is that of the *balneum cinereum* or "ash bath," which is made by burying the bottom of the vessel in another containing hot ashes. This fire is anodyne, mild, slightly dry, and temperate in

---

*[The Egyptian alchemist Mary the Jewess is widely credited with the invention of the water bath or bain-marie, which still bears her name to this day; see Marcellin Berthelot, *Les origines de l'alchimie,* 56. —*Trans.*]

nature. It is suitable for certain digestions, circulations, distillations, and slow coagulations.

4. The fourth fire is that of the *balneum siccum* or "sand bath," which is made by burying the bottom of the vessel in another containing hot sand. This fire is dry and moderately hot. It is used for distillation and coagulation.
5. The fifth fire is a variation of *balneum arenae* that uses iron filings instead of ash or sand, with the iron filings interposed between the coal fire and the vessel. This fire is hot and dry. It is suitable for violent distillations and certain sublimations.
6. The sixth fire is the *coal fire,* which is made in a closed reverberatory to extract certain spirits. This fire is used primarily in sublimations.
7. The seventh fire is the *fire of fusion,* which is made with dry wood and coal. This fire is suitable for calcinations, sublimations, carburations, reverberations, and vitrifications.

Each of these fires is divided into various degrees: the steam bath, the water bath, the ash bath, and the sand bath each have three degrees, and the other fires each have four degrees. Numerous works of premodern chemistry give ample descriptions of the furnaces and apparatuses necessary for basic chemical operations. Among these works, those of Johann Rudolf Glauber, Nicolas Lémery, and Antoine Baumé are serviceable and readily accessible.[1] It would be appropriate, however, to say a few words about vessels.

The Vessels of Premodern Chemistry

Glass vessels are best, but they are suitable only for steam, water, or sand baths. Metallic vessels are necessary for the more violent fires and for large quantities of plant matter. Corrosive substances such as salts, vitriols, or acids require vessels made of glass or glazed earth. The following are the most commonly used vessels:

🌿 The **glass cucurbit** covered with its head or cap is suitable for basic distillations of plants over a soft fire.

🌿 The ***copper bladder*** tinned on the inside and equipped with a Moor's head is necessary for distillations of large quantities.*

🌿 The ***tin campana*** or bell-shaped vessel adapted to a large basin of copper is used for distillations of fresh fruits, flowers, and succulents.

🌿 The ***retort*** equipped with a large container or glass balloon serves for the distillation *per latus* of oils and spirits that are too heavy to ascend.

🌿 The ***copper alembic*** lined with tin or the still head with its refrigeratory is used for other distillations. It consists of a serpentine or spiral tube adapted to a receiver.

🌿 The ***long-necked matrass*** and the ***circulatory vessel*** made of two matrasses or cucurbits luted together are suitable for digestions over a slow fire (*ignis lentus*).

🌿 The single or twin ***pelican*** is suitable for circulation.

🌿 The ***aludel,*** the ***blind alembic,*** or the ***inverted crucible*** is required for sublimations.

🌿 Finally, the ***crucible of refractory earth*** is suitable for the fire of fusion.

Decoction and Infusion

The operations of decoction and infusion serve the same purpose, which is to dissolve and extract the active principles from bodies in a vehicle well suited to the intended purpose. Decoction, however, differs from infusion in that it involves more extraneous principles and is performed in the open air and in an open vessel, the contents of which are brought to a boil. This operation does not preserve the volatile parts of the material. The quantity of the vehicle to be added to the plant matter is relative to its volume and to the duration of boiling, which is longer for more compact substances such as guaiac wood, Indian bulrush, and other woods and hard roots.

---

*[The so-called Moor's head, a name which recalls its Islamic origins, is a copper cap that is tinned on the inside and fashioned in the shape of a head. It surrounds the alembic (or still head) and is filled with cold water in order to achieve a more efficient condensation of the distilling vapors. —*Trans.*]

In some cases, decoction must be preceded by infusion. Aromatic plants should not be boiled, however, for their virtue lies in their volatile principle, which the heat causes to evaporate through the opening of the vessel. It is necessary, then, to *infuse* such plants in a closed vessel and then to *filter* the liquor only after it has cooled down inside the vessel. The purpose of infusion is to extract the subtlest soluble parts from mixed bodies by means of an appropriate menstruum or solvent, which is why boiling is prohibited in this operation.

The various menstrua necessary for infusions are wine, vinegar, alcohol, and sometimes mineral spirits. These vehicles must be imbued with the virtue of the mixed bodies they bathe and penetrate, to the point that their own nature is attenuated. The practitioner must avoid mixing the water contained in the residue with the liquor extracted, because this water is impure. The residue, however, can be calcined to extract the fixed salt, which may then be dissolved in its liquor.

Spagyric infusion is markedly different from vulgar infusion, and this difference lies especially in the nature of the menstrua, which we shall discuss in due course.

Digestion and Distillation

Digestion and distillation are among the most important spagyric operations. Digestion or circulation consists in cooking the material by the heat of water so that the humidity intervenes in a temperate mode of hot and dry qualities, causing a slow digestion that gradually alters the material, separates its parts, and forces its molecules toward a profitable evolution in the distillatory process. Distillation consists in extracting the liquid and volatile parts in which the spirit possessing the virtue of the mixed body resides.

The operative procedures will vary according to the nature of the material and the aim of the operator. Sometimes herbalists will need to reduce the plant matter down to five separate principles; other times they will need to extract only one of these principles. With jalap, for example, it is sufficient to extract the resinous substance alone and disregard the other principles. Likewise, the herbalist may extract the essential oil of anise by distillation and ignore the remaining substances, and so on.

Whichever whole plants or plant parts one chooses to distill should be grated, chopped into fine pieces, or powderized so that they may be introduced more easily into a retort, and this should be done with water *if they are dry* but without water *if they are fresh.*

When the retort is set over the fire, first the phlegm, then the spirit, and then the oil will pour out into the receiver, while the fixed salt will remain in the residue that collects at the bottom of the retort. This residue may be calcined and the fixed salt extracted by lixiviation and evaporation. The salt may then be dissolved in the spirit to increase its virtue. Moist vegetal matter like must and other saps should be distilled with the alembic in the sand bath prior to fermentation. Again, first the phlegm, then the spirit, and then the oil will pour out into the receiver, while the earth will remain at the bottom. In distillations of wine, however, the spirit will ascend first.

Thus, in order to extract the five principles from fermented liquors such as wine, beer, cider, and mead, they must be distilled first over a slow fire and the heat should be increased only gradually. In this case, the subtle and inflammable spirit will ascend first, then the water, and then the oily empyreumatic spirit, and the salt and earth will remain at the bottom. Liquors whose fermentations are advanced to a sort of corruption such as vinegar and all very sour waters will release their water first, then their acid spirit, and lastly their stinking oil. Having thus destroyed the form of these mixed bodies, each principle may be separated using the following procedures: the oil will separate from its spirit and phlegm by funneling; the spirit will separate from its phlegm by rectification; and the salt will separate from its dead earth by calcination and depuration.

Our purpose here is not to reinvent the wheel and provide an exhaustive study of the basic principles of premodern chemistry. There are numerous detailed and readily accessible studies on this subject. However, in order to clarify this study perfectly, we shall focus here on the chemical preparations of plants and describe in detail the operations of one particularly skillful pharmaceutical chemist, Christophe Glaser. Although Glaser's operations fall somewhat outside the scope of our main subject, we include them here for the benefit of students, and beginners especially.

The various products discovered by analyses of various plant compositions are not equally distributed throughout their being. This distribution varies according to their species, and a consideration of these differences implies the need for different preparations. Glaser follows Ettmüller's classification of plants and describes the simplest and best preparations for each class according to the methods of ordinary chemistry. His lessons also have the advantage of being adaptable to a great number of different cases.

The reader should note that all of the recipes in this book make use of old weights and measures, and that all measurements in pounds are weighted according to the old *medicinal pound* (see Table 12.1 on page 107).

General Preparation of Leaves:
Preparing Lettuces and Plants of Ettmüller's 1st Class

Lettuces should be picked when their leaves are full of juice and ready to shoot up into stalks. Beat a good amount of lettuce in a mortar and press out the juice. Let it stand for two or three hours and pour the clearest liquid into a glass cucurbit. Approximately one-third of the lettuce juice should remain, which is unsuitable for distillation but can be used for other purposes. Distill the juice in the cucurbit, which is the best choice of vessel, and clarify it by filtration or by passing it through a cloth strainer. Evaporate the liquid until it becomes as thick as honey, and add a little sugar or salt if you wish to preserve it.

The thick syrup must be dissolved in its own water. Its dose is from 1 to 2 drams in 5 to 6 ounces of its own water.[2] This soporific julep is refreshing, tempers the heat of the bile, and moderates all humoral irritations.

Distillation of Succulent Herbs,
Lettuces, and Plants of Ettmüller's 1st Class

For this operation use a broad and flat tinned copper cauldron and set upon it an alembic made of tin rather than lead. Put the herbs or leaves in the copper cauldron and fit it into a larger iron cauldron filled with an inch and a half of sand.

Cover the copper cauldron with its dome-shaped head or a cap of fine tin and adapt it to a receiver. Stoke the fire little by little, increasing the heat gradually until the water distills drop by drop. Maintain the same degree of heat until the moisture of the leaves evaporates and condenses into water and the leaves become so dry and arid that they may be powderized. The water extracted will be imbued with the virtue of the leaves, which would have burned off were it not protected by sand from the violent action of the fire.

This operation is suitable not only for succulent herbs devoid of acid, but also for flowers such as roses, lilies, water lilies, opium poppies, common poppies, and others. If the remaining herbs are burned to ashes, their salt can be extracted by washing, provided the herbs remain whole, as their leaves alone are devoid of salt.[3]

Distillation of Sorrel and Plants of Ettmüller's 2nd Class

It is necessary first to separate the water and the acid salt from these plants. Take a good amount of sorrel and draw the juice by expression, then let it settle for twelve hours. Decant the clear liquid into one or more glass cucurbits, then distill off about two-thirds in the bain-marie and save the water. Filter the juice through a cloth strainer to purify it, then filter the juice that remains at the bottom of the cucurbits by passing it through a cloth strainer.

Transfer the juice to another, larger cucurbit and finish drawing out the phlegm in the bain-marie until it reaches the consistency of a thick syrup. Store the cucurbit in the cellar for a few days, after which time a portion of the juice will have converted into a salt similar to tartar. Decant the supernating liquor and dry the essential salt. Return it to the cellar once more and allow this liquor to continue evaporating. Part of it will form into salt, which should be added to the first salt. To purify the salt, dissolve it in its own distilled water, then filter it. Allow it to evaporate and crystallize as before and you will obtain the essential salt.

This essential salt, which contains the principal virtue of the sorrel, opens obstructions of the liver and the spleen, reverses corruption, and refreshes and arouses the appetite by fortifying the stomach. It is also febrifugal and antibilious. Its dose is from 20 grains to 1 dram dissolved in its own water.[4]

Distillation of Blessed Thistle and Plants of Ettmüller's 3rd Class

These odorless plants have a bitter and biting taste and contain high levels of water and nitrous essential salt.

Take a good amount of blessed thistle when it is ready to shoot out its stalk, draw out the juice by expression as in the previous example, and let it settle for several hours. Distill as before to draw out the salutary water. The juice remaining in the bottom of the cucurbits must be clarified and evaporated to the consistency of an extract. If you want to make an essential salt, which will have a nitrous taste, proceed as directed in the previous example concerning the sorrel juice. It is better, however, to purify it by dissolving it in its own distilled water and to filter it through a brown paper filter in which you have put some ashes of the blessed thistle. Next, evaporate it until a film rises on the top and you will obtain a salt similar to saltpeter and a fuel that burns like saltpeter. To extract only the blessed thistle's water, distill the leaves in the sand bath using a cauldron similar to the one described above, and you will obtain an excellent water possessing a greater virtue than that of the water extracted by the water bath.

The essential salt serves as an excellent remedy for hot fevers and infectious diseases, as it removes toxins through perspiration. Its dose is from 6 to 12 grains.[5]

Distillation of Watercress and Plants of the Ettmüller's 4th Class

These plants contain high levels of sulfurous and volatile essential salt and may be distilled and reduced into an extract or essential salt in the same manner as plants of the preceding class. But their principal virtue resides in their spirituous and hot substance, which can be extracted using the following method:

Harvest a large quantity of watercress (approximately 40 pounds) as soon as it begins to bloom and before its seed appears. Cut the watercress into small pieces and grind them in a marble mortar, then transfer them in this state to a barrel that is open on one side only and pour hot (but not scalding) water over the watercress up to twice the apparent volume of the leaves.

Stir well with a mixing stick, then cover the open side of the barrel with cloth sheets to preserve the volatile spirits and let it sit for half an hour or more. Next, add three times the amount of water that was first poured in, but less hot, so that there is eight times as much water as plant matter. Then add 3 or 4 pounds of yeast and stir well with a mixing stick. Tightly cover the barrel, which should be more than half full, and set it in a temperate place (a bit warmer than cold). In three or four days the coarse substance will rise above the liquor in the form of a crust, which will be ready for distillation as soon as it begins to break and sag. At this moment, set everything in a large copper bladder tinned on the inside to distill the *aqua vitae*. Distill out the spirit, which will be mixed with water, starting with a gradual and gentle fire, then rectify the spirit using the same vessel. When deprived of all its phlegm, the spirit will be pure and flammable.

This spirit is effective against scurvy and corruptions of the blood. Its penetrating virtue resolves, purifies, and subtilizes all impure humors. Its dose is from 20 grains to 1 dram in a suitable vehicle.[6]

Distillation of Wormwood and Plants of the Ettmüller's 5th Class

These plants can be fermented in the same manner as watercress and plants of Ettmüller's 4th class, but their principal virtue resides in the sulfurous and subtle substance that floats on its water, which may be extracted using the following procedure:

Harvest a large quantity of wormwood tops when they are *between flower and seed*. Cut them into small pieces and grind them in a marble mortar, then transfer them to a tinned copper bladder and pour in enough water to saturate all of the wormwood. The vessel should be no more than half-full and covered with a Moor's head. Gradually increase the heat of the fire until the drops begin to fall, then raise the heat until the drops succeed each other rapidly and continue in this manner until the water that comes out is insipid. The receiver will contain an abundance of spirituous water, upon which the oil will float. Separate the oil in the following manner: fill the receiver up to the rim and attach a small vial to its neck with a string, then introduce a small cotton wick into the hole of the vial and dip the other end into the oil floating on the surface of the water in the receiver. The wick will attract and soak up the oil, which will drip into and fill up the vial. If the water decreases, refill the receiver so that the oil is always high and reaches the rim of the container. Continue until all of the oil has been separated and store it in a well-stopped vial.

The oils contain all the virtue of these balsamic plants. Do not discard the distilled waters after separating the oils, however, as they may be preserved and used later for other purposes.[7]

TABLE 12.1.

OLD WEIGHTS AND MEASURES AND THEIR EQUIVALENTS

Old Weights	Equivalences	Weights in grams
Medicinal pound	12 ounces	367 grams
Merchant pound	16 ounces or 2 dregs	489 grams
Half pound	6 or 8 ounces	186 or 245 grams
Ounce	8 drams	30.59 grams
Half ounce or lot	4 drams	15.30 grams
Dram	3 scruples	3.82 grams
Half dram	36 grains	1.91 grams
Scruple	24 grains	1.27 grams
Grain		0.05 grams

13
Plant Juices and Their Uses

By "juice" we refer to the liquors contained in vegetables, which are composed of various substances such as salts, oils, gums, resins, and milks. These juices can be extracted depending on the nature of the plant by *maceration* or by *expression*. They are divisible into three main classes:

1st Class: aqueous and watery juices.

2nd Class: oily, resinous, essential, and unctuous juices.

3rd Class: milky, mucilaginous, and emulsive juices.

To extract the juice from a plant, first pick it while it is fresh, then wash, drain, and chop it roughly, and pound it in a marble mortar until it is sufficiently crushed. Enclose it in a muslin bag and express its juice by means of a special press made for this purpose. The juice will escape little by little and be clouded by some of the plant particles it carries with it.

For plants with thick and mucilaginous juices such as borage, bugloss, and chicory, it is necessary to add a little water when pounding them and to let them macerate a few hours prior to expression, but aromatic plants should never undergo maceration. The process is the same for roots, too, only sometimes they will need to be grated due to their viscosity. Plants that render their water most easily are those that are soft, sweet, and cold such as salads, houseleeks, fruits, gourds, lemons, oranges, and barberries, among others.

Once the juice of a plant has been extracted, it needs to be clarified.

To do so, fill three-quarters of a matrass with the juice and immerse the matrass in near boiling water. Remove the matrass occasionally so that it heats gradually and the parenchyma clots in the liquid. When the liquid cools down, strain it to filter out the parenchymal lumps. Some juices such as houseleek, cucumber, lemon, currant, barberry, and cherry will clarify naturally without any preparation. Just bottle them, let them settle, and filter them. To preserve these juices, bottle them after a perfect clarification. Pour a little olive oil on top, then hermetically seal the bottle and store it in a cool place.

To obtain the salts contained in plant juices, evaporate them until they reach the consistency of a syrup. Store the syrup in a cool place protected from dust, and in fifteen to thirty days crystals will form on the surface. Remove the crystals and keep them in tightly sealed jars. These salts, which possess the virtue of the plants from which they have been extracted, are resolutive and sometimes depurative.

Treatment of Seeds

Seeds must be prepared differently according to their substance. Some are mucilaginous, like quince, flax, and psyllium seeds, while others are filled with oils that can be drawn by expression and reduced to an emulsion, such as peony, poppy, fiber hemp, and the greater and lesser cold seeds. From some seeds, like mustard and pepper, one can extract a fiery spirit by fermentation, while others are aromatic and contain a sulfur or an ethereal and subtle oil, like caraway, anise, and fennel seeds, which may be distilled in the same manner as wormwood and juniper berries. This oil, however, must be separated from the water immediately after distillation, because otherwise they will mix together.[1]

Almost all seeds distilled by the retort will leave a quantity of volatile salt attached to the walls of the vessel. When this salt is dissolved in its own oil, it will increase the oil's virtue. All these seeds will render their oil by distillation, but their oil must be separated from their water using the method indicated above for distillations of wormwood and plants of Ettmüller's 5th class. But seed oils can also be extracted by expression, as we shall demonstrate.

Anise Seed Oil Extracted by Expression

Finely pulverize 1 pound of anise seed and put it on an inverted sieve covered with a tin dish so that all the anise seed is contained under the cap of the dish. Set the sieve in a flat basin containing 2 or 3 pints of water. Set it on the fire and bring the water to a boil. The water vapor will penetrate the anise seed. When the tin dish that covers the anise becomes exceedingly hot, transfer the powder into a canvas bag and bind it promptly. Then place it in a heated press and extract the oil, which will have a strong aroma and a very pronounced flavor.[2]

The Cox Method of Plant Preparation

Gather in warm weather a considerable quantity of the leaves of any plant, stripped or pulled from the greater stalks. Press the leaves tightly together in several heaps and let the process of fermentation run its course. The leaves will resolve into a pappy substance, except for the outer leaves, which must be removed and discarded. Form this substance into pellets and put them in a glass retort, then distill, ending with a high heat. Besides a great quantity of liquor, they will yield a thick black oil of a balsamic consistence. Separate the liquor from the oil, then distill it in a glass cucurbit and it will raise a volatile spirit which, after two or three rectifications, will have the taste and smell of sal ammoniac.[3]

Using this method, plants that render good quantities of fixed salt like wormwood, sage, and rosemary will render like quantities of volatile salt, which should be dissolved in the distilled spirit already obtained. We should note, however, that this method of preparation is vulgar rather than spagyric.

Reduction of Guaiac Wood into Five Different Substances

This curious operation is particularly enlightening with regard to the chemical division of all plants.

Put 4 pounds of grated guaiac wood in a well-luted retort made of sandstone or glass, set it in the closed reverberatory furnace, and fit it to a large receiver without luting. Increase the fire gradually and it will render first an insipid water and then a volatile spirit having an intense flavor. As soon as the spirit ascends, empty the water from the receiver and keep it in another vessel, then join the receiver and the retort and lute the joints carefully. Since these spirits are violent, maintain a moderate fire for seven or eight hours, then increase it little by little, and continue for as long as the spirit and the oil issue out together. The spirit and the oil can be separated easily. Just pour the entire contents of the receiver into a funnel lined with filter paper and place it over a vial. The spirit will pass through, and the oil will remain. Place the funnel over another vial, make a hole in the paper filter for the oil to flow through, and preserve it separately. Reduce the wood remaining in the retort to ashes and extract the salt by washing, filtering, and evaporating.

The spirit heals cankers, ulcers, fistulas, and corrupt wounds. It has a biting taste, but this can be tempered with its water. When rectified in the water bath, it flushes out toxins and viruses through the urine and sweat. Its dose is from 20 drops to 1 dram in a specific decoction. The oil can be rectified using the ash bath, but it will lose some of its virtue. The oil is good for epilepsy, soothes toothaches, reabsorbs hemorrhoids, and dries fistulas. Its dose is from 3 to 6 drops in a liquor. Juniper, boxwood, and linden woods can be treated in the same manner.[4]

Preparations of Juniper Berries

These preparations are designed to draw the fiery spirit of juniper berries by distillation and to extract the ethereal oil and the medicinal extract known as "German Treacle."* The ardent spirit is the product of fermentation, which is performed with warm water and beer yeast as in the previous example concerning watercress and plants of Ettmüller's 4th class. The distillation should take place only after the process of fermentation is complete. This operation is not applicable to all berries, however, because those of the elder and the dwarf elder,

---

*[The French "thériaque des Allemands" and its English equivalent "German Treacle" are old pharmaceutical names for "medicinal gin." See Louis Chambaud, *The Idioms of the French and English Languages,* 6. Like a great many other liquors, gin has its origins in herbal medicine. —*Trans.*]

among others, will ferment without any additives in the same manner as grapes, apples, and pears. These should be sufficiently crushed and stored for eight to ten days in a large vessel. Once they have finished fermenting, the time will be ripe to distill the fiery spirit, which has great virtues. Use the following procedure to distill the ethereal oil:

Crush 6 pounds of juniper berries and place them in a copper bladder, pour over 50 pounds of common water, stir everything together, and cover the bladder with a Moor's head. Distill the spirituous water and oil, which will come out together, with a gradual fire and continue until the water that emerges becomes insipid. Next, separate the oil from the water as instructed in the above preparation of wormwood and store these two liquids separately in well-sealed vials. Remove what remains in the bottom of the bladder while it is still warm and put it in several terrines, then pass it through a cloth filter to express the marc. Let the liquor rest for fifteen hours, then pass the clear liquid through a fine cloth filter and evaporate the filtered liquor to the consistency of an extract.

Both the spirit and the oil are powerful herbal remedies for provoking menstruation, opening obstructions of the liver and the spleen, and breaking up stones and phlegm in the kidneys and the bladder. They are powerful sudorifics and stimulate urination. The dose of the spirit is from ½ dram to 1 tablespoon in a lettuce broth. The dose of the oil is from 3 to 15 drops in its own water. The dose of the extract is from 1 to 3 drams in its own water.[5]

Jalap Root Extract

The root of the jalap, which is native to the Indies, should be heavy and gray-black in color. Its chief virtue resides in the resin, which may be extracted using the following procedure:

Put 8 ounces of pulverized jalap root in a matrass and pour over four fingers of a good spirit of wine. Stop the matrass and set it to digest in the bain-marie for two or three days, during which time the spirit will turn hyacinthine in color. Decant the colored spirit into another vessel and pour a new spirit of wine over the matter and set it to digest as before. This must be done three times in all. Mix the three spirits together, then filter and pour them into a large glazed terrine with 3 or 4 pounds of pure water, and let the jalap root precipitate to the bottom. Pour off the water into a cucurbit and remove the spirit by distillation. Wash the resin with clean water, dry it in the Sun, and pulverize it before using it.

This resin purges serosities and flushes out phlegms and aqueous humors. Its dose is from 5 to 15 grains in a bolus-shaped extract or with vitriolated tartar powder or, even better, diluted in an emulsion of cold seeds. The resins of scammony, agaric, and turpeth may also be prepared using this method.[6]

Black Hellebore Root Extract

This preparation can serve as a model for all roots that contain a water-soluble juice such as mechoacan (the white tuberous root of the largeroot morning glory) and leafy spurge, wild cucumber, and rhubarb roots, among others.

Grind 1 pound of young and fresh black hellebore root and transfer it to a cucurbit with 5 or 6 pounds of distilled rainwater. Cover the cucurbit with a blind alembic and set it to digest in a hot sand bath for two days. When the two days are up, pass the liquor through a linen filter and express the marc a little, over which it will be necessary to pour more fresh water and then digest as before. Pour out this liquor and mix it with the other. Filter the mixture, then evaporate it in a terrine until it thickens and store it in a tightly sealed jar.

This extract is good for melancholic diseases. Its dose is from 12 to 30 grains in any vegetable broth.[7]

Angelica Root Extract

Put 1 pound of ground angelica root in a cucurbit and pour over 6 pounds of good white wine or weak brandy. Cover the cucurbit with a blind alembic and set it to digest in the steam bath for two or three days. Remove the blind alembic and replace it with a beak alembic, adapt it to a receiver, and lute the joints well. Begin distilling in the water bath and continue until you have drawn off 3 pounds of water, which will contain the volatile principle of the angelica root. Keep this water in a well-sealed vessel. Allow the vessels to cool, then strain and strongly express what remains in the cucurbit and pass the liquor through a filter to clarify it. Evaporate it in the gentle heat of the bain-marie in a terrine until it reaches the consistency of an extract. Calcine the marc left over from the expression and reduce it to ashes, making a lye, then filter and evaporate it into salt. Mix the salt with the extract and preserve them together in a well-sealed vessel.

This extract is aperitive and diaphoretic. It causes sweating, provokes menstruation, combats suffocations of the womb, counters venoms and toxins, and destroys infectious and contagious diseases. Its dose is from 10 to 30 grains in its own water, which is also very effective by itself. The same procedure may be used to draw the water, extract, and salt from all roots that contain a sulfurous and volatile salt, and have both an aromatic odor and a warm flavor, such as valerian, wild angelica, spignel, carline thistle, sweet flag, zedoary, and galangal roots.[8]

Spirit and Oil of Angelica Root

To obtain this spirit, grind the roots and digest them with a good quantity of distilled water and a little spirit of wine for four full days in the water bath. Next, put everything in a tinned copper bladder over a graduated fire until the spirits ascend, then subject it to a stronger, continuous, and regulated fire until the spirituous water comes out, which you will recognize by its insipid flavor.

To separate the spirit from the water, rectify it slowly in the water bath and you will obtain a subtle spirit full of a volatile salt. This spirit serves as a diaphoretic and diuretic alexitary. Its virtue counters all infectious diseases and afflictions of the womb. Its dose is from ½ scruple to 1 dram either in its own water or in a vegetable broth.

The oil of angelica root will float on the surface of the water of the first distillation made in the copper bladder. Separate it using a cotton wick as instructed in the preparation of wormwood and carefully preserve it. This oil prevents the onset of all infectious and contagious diseases. The oil can then be treated in the same manner as nutmeg.

Spirit, Oil, and Balm of Nutmeg

Oil of nutmeg may be extracted by expression using the normal method:

Put 4 ounces of pure nutmeg oil in a long-necked matrass, add four fingers of tartarized spirit of wine, and set it to digest in the water bath with a slow heat. Decant the spirit as soon as it is dyed and resume the operation with another spirit until it no longer draws a dye. Wash the residue in a bowl with boiling water until the mass becomes odorless and white—this is the body of the balm, which can be colored by cooking it with an inodorous and neutral plant. To prepare this balm and give it the necessary virtue, mix it with its aromatic oil until it forms into a creamy balm.

As for the nutmeg oil mixed with the tartarized spirit of wine, distill it in the bain-marie until it reaches the consistency of honey in order to extract the spirit. In this manner you will obtain a nutmeg extract filled with the best of its intimate essence and a spirit endowed with its oil and volatile salt. These remedies are good for the stomach, the brain, and the womb. They dispel flatulence, promote digestion, correct bad breath, strengthen the embryo, and heal syncope, palpitations, and obstructions.

Distillation of Cinnamon Bark

This preparation can serve as a model for aromatic barks such as lemon and orange bark, as well as for nutmeg, clove, and pepper, among other herbs.

Grind 4 pounds of red cinnamon into a coarse powder, which should have a strong and sweet aroma and a pungent and astringent taste, and place it in a sandstone jar. Pour in 12 pounds of rainwater, add ½ pound of saltpeter, and let it macerate for four days. Next, empty all the material into a tinned copper bladder and add an additional 12 pounds of fresh water. Place the bladder in the reverberatory furnace, adapt its refrigeratory and receiver, and lute the joints well. Maintain from the start a medium fire, so that the drops succeed each other without interruption and the oil and spirit ascend together. Continue this step until the water that comes out is devoid of strength. Be sure to refresh the water in the refrigeratory every so often, the better to condense the spirits. When the distillation is complete, separate the water from the oil, which will settle at the bottom of the receiver in a very small quantity. This oil contains the principal virtue of the cinnamon. If you want this highly concentrated oil to mix more easily with liquors, mix it with some powdered sugar.

This refreshing oil provokes menstruation, promotes digestion, and strengthens the stomach and the womb. Its dose is ½ drop in some liquor. Its water has the same properties but is less effective (its dose is 1 or 2 tablespoons).[9]

Tincture of Cinnamon

Put 4 ounces of ground cinnamon in a matrass and pour over 1 pound of good spirit of wine. Adapt another matrass to the first, making a well-luted circulatory vessel. Set it to digest with a slow heat for three or four days, after which time the spirit will turn red. Then decant, filter, and store the tincture in a well-stopped vial.

The tincture has almost the same virtues as the oil. Its dose is ½ tablespoon in a suitable liquor. When the tincture is reduced by distillation, its virtue is greatly increased.[10]

Sublimation of Benzoin Flowers

Put 4 ounces of good benzoin in a glazed earthenware pot with a rim and fit it with a paper cornet. The cornet should be well-glued and measure one foot high; its opening should be measured to the size of the rim of the pot. Fasten the two together with a loop of string. Place the pot in the sand bath for half an hour, then loosen the cornet to remove the flowers that have accumulated on it and replace the cornet immediately with another previously measured and prepared. Continue and repeat this procedure every half hour until the flowers become charged with oil. Then stop the fire and carefully preserve the flowers in a well-sealed jar.

Transfer what remains in the pot into a glass retort and distill it in the sand bath with a gradual heat. A thick and fragrant oil will come out that is excellent for wounds and ulcers. The flowers are good for bronchial and pulmonary pain and for asthma. Its dose is 4 to 6 grains in a sweet tart dough or jam.[11]

Preparation of Aloe

Put ½ pound of Fybnos aloe in a glass cucurbit and pour over 1½ pounds of violet juice. Cover the cucurbit with the blind alembic and set it to digest for forty-eight hours. When the aloe is dissolved, decant and filter the liquid, then evaporate it in a bowl in the steam bath to reduce it into a mass. From this mass or *aloes violata,* make pills weighing 6 or 8 grains apiece.

Its dose is one pill before supper. The aloe is hepatic, antibilious, and vermifugal. It also fortifies the stomach.[12]

Preparation of Opium

Opium is the concentrated juice of the opium poppy. The juice is drawn by incising the poppy heads shortly before their maturity, which is preferable to drawing the juice from the whole plant by expression.

Cut this brown and glossy resin into thin slices, spread them out in a glazed earthenware dish, and place it on a small coal fire. Stir the opium frequently, which will first soften and then solidify. Continue the fire until the material crumbles between the fingers, and take care to avoid the noxious fumes. Put the roasted opium in a matrass and pour over four fingers of distilled dew water, then stop the matrass and set it to digest in the water bath for four days. The water will turn a reddish-brown color. Pour this tincture into another vessel, then pour more dew water over the matter to complete the extraction of the tincture. Filter the whole mixture and evaporate it in the water bath until it reaches the consistency of an extract.

Opium when prepared in this manner has the virtue of appeasing the nerves and arresting diarrhea. It promotes sleep and softens acrimonious humors. Its dose is from ½ to 2 grains. In the absence of dew water, use distilled rainwater.[13]

Observation on the Distillation of Common Centaury, Wormwood, Rue, Lemon Balm, Mint, Valerian, Linden Flower, and All Plants Whose Nature is Dry and Balsamic

All these plants should to be cut into pieces and roughly ground in a mortar. Add 10 pounds of water for each pound of plant matter and, if you wish to ferment and distill them to extract the spirit, proceed as directed in the preceding chapter. But if it is simply a matter of distilling the ethereal oil and the spirituous water, then it is only necessary to distill them after they have been chopped and cut into very fine pieces with 10 pounds of water per pound of plant matter, without prior infusion, maceration, or fermentation.

The Medicinal Virtues of *Nostoc* or *Flos coeli*

Nostoc or *flos coeli,* according to Quesnot, is nothing more than a vapor that issues from the earth during the time of the equinoxes, from March 20 to April 21 and from September 21 to October 22.* It comes bubbling out of the ground before sunrise in the form of a thick sap that has the smell of sulfur and takes on various forms according to the nature of the earth. It coagulates in the form of a transparent emeraldine glass, which some philosophers call "vitriol" (*vitri-oleum*) in order to hide its true identity. These large, thin sheets or "leaves" are more readily found in sandy areas. They should be gathered in places exposed to the rising Sun, but just before sunrise, because the Sun's heat volatilizes them.[14] Here is its preparation:

Once gathered, gently wash the *Nostoc* in fountain water and wipe it gently, then spread it on a white cloth and let it dry overnight. Grind it in a mortar, then put it in a well-luted glass vessel and let it sit buried in the sand for forty days without fire. At the end of the philosophical month, pass it through a press to extract the blood-colored liquor into which it resolved over the last forty days. Pour this

---

*[The term *Nostoc,* first coined by Paracelsus, is the modern genus name for several species of cyanobacteria now known by the common names "troll's butter," "witch's jelly," and "star jelly," the latter comparable to Quesnot's *flos coeli,* which means "flower of heaven." —*Trans.*]

liquor into a glass alembic until it is half full, adapt it to a receiver of the same dimensions, and lute the joints well. Expose it to the air, to the day, to the night, and to the celestial influences, and the water will distill all by itself, becoming clear and limpid, in a quantity ten times smaller than the original amount of liquor. This distillation should last approximately forty days.

This water, Quesnot asserts, is an anodyne and invigorating universal solvent that can break up gallstones. To make a great arcanum, cook it in a closed matrass in the water bath. The matrass should be joined with another to make a circulatory vessel, but the pelican would be even better. Over the course of this slow circulation, the matter will cohobate on its own and eventually freeze in a crystalline form. It is also possible to proceed by slow distillation, by cohobating the spirit on its residue seven times, but this procedure takes more time and is less profitable.

The crystals will divide on their own and should be preserved in a sealed jar. This powder contains within itself the ethereal virtue of all living substances and is particularly beneficial for the preservation of our natural heat and radical moisture. Quesnot claims that this is the true Mercury of the Philosophers and the natural solvent of gold, but this is an opinion we do not share.

14

Le Fèvre's Chemical Preparations of Plants

Preparation of Succulent Nitrous Plants

Take a large quantity of a succulent nitrous plant such as eastern pellitory-of-the-wall, fumitory, purslane, borage, bugloss, mercury, or nightshade and beat it in parcels in a marble mortar to reduce it to a pulp. Express the pulp in a bag of horsehair, muslin, or cloth and strain the juice through a Hippocrates's sleeve. Let it settle so that it leaves its sediment behind and gently decant it into glass cucurbits. To obtain a good extract and a soft water, use the water bath, because the heat of the water bath is not strong enough to elevate the essential nitrous salt and causes it to remain mixed with the thickened juice or extract at the bottom of the vessel. But to obtain a strong water (*aqua fortis*) animated by this spirituous salt that can be preserved for a long time, put the cucurbits in the sand bath, because this fire will elevate and volatilize the most subtle part of the salt and cause it to rise along with the water vapor near the end of the distillation. But take care that the heat is not too violent near the end of the distillation so that it does not overly dry out the residue at the bottom of the vessel, and before the operation's conclusion be sure to clarify the juice completely by passing the purified juice once more through a Hippocrates's sleeve.

Once the juice has been purified, continue the distillation with the same type of fire chosen at the beginning of the operation until the juice reduces to a syrup, then store it in the cellar or in a cool place until the essential nitro-tartarous salt crystallizes and separates from the juice. Next, decant the juice slowly, return it to the water or sand bath, and evaporate it until it reaches the consistency of an extract, which, if cooked in the water bath, will still contain a lot of salt and be useful for making opiates or other remedies, depending on the nature of the plant in question. In this manner you will obtain the distilled water, the purified juice in the form of an extract, and the essential salt.

To prepare the fixed salt, dry the pomace or residue remaining after the expression of the juice and calcine it to a light ash, then leach it with rainwater or fountain water and filter it through some scotch paper, lightly glued, so that the liquor passes through in a short amount of time. Once you have extracted the first salt, leach the marc with fresh water to extract the remainder of the salt. Repeat this procedure until the water becomes tasteless.

After mixing all the filtered lyes together, evaporate them in earthenware bowls in the sand bath until they thicken to a film, then gently agitate the liquor with a spatula until the salt is sufficiently dried. Put this salt in a crucible and reverberate it in the wind furnace until it turns red, but without melting it. Remove the crucible from the fire, let it cool, then dissolve the salt in the water extracted from the plant and filter it once more. Put this dissolved salt in a glass cucurbit equipped with an alembic and redraw the water from the salt using the sand bath until it thickens to a film, then remove it from the fire and let it crystallize in a cool place. Continue these operations until all of the salt is extracted.

When mixed with the water drawn from the plant, this purified salt becomes not only more active and efficacious, but also more durable. It can be preserved for several years without losing any of its virtue. The proportion of the mixture is 2 drams of salt to 1 pint of water. The salt serves as a mild laxative. It provokes urination and opens obstructions of the lower parts of the body, but its chief virtue depends on the nature of the plant from which it was extracted.

The nitro-tartarous salts can be purified by several dissolutions in common water. Pour this water on the ashes of the plant and evaporate it in a terrine in the sand bath. Continue until two-thirds of the water has evaporated, but not so long that it develops a film, and pour the remaining third while it is still hot into another terrine without disturbing the bottom. Remove the water that floats above the crystals and repeat the evaporation until the water reduces by half. Continue until all of the salt has crystallized.[1]

Preparation of Succulents Containing a Volatile Essential Salt

The preparation of succulent plants that contain a volatile essential salt and have an acrid, pungent, and aromatic taste such as watercress, stone parsley, hedge mustard, arugula, water parsnip, scurvy grass, mustard, and horseradish differs little from the preparation of the nitro-tartarous plants described above.

This operation requires special attention, however, because if it is prolonged for too long, the volatile and subtle saline spirit will dissipate from the heat and take the virtue of the plant along with it. These plants should be picked when they have recently sprouted and have begun to form the umbels of their flowers because this is the very moment when their essential salt is exalted. As for the rest of the procedure, follow the directions of the previous operation, but do not put the essential volatile salt in the crucible, because it will evaporate.[2]

Extracting Spirits from Succulents Containing a Volatile Essential Salt

Take a certain quantity of one of these plants, remove any dead leaves, and clean it thoroughly. Bruise it in parcels in a marble mortar and transfer them immediately to a large glass matrass or balloon. Pour over hot water up to the height of half a foot, then stop the neck of the matrass with the blind alembic (or adapt another matrass to make a circulatory vessel). Let it rest for two hours, then add fresh lukewarm water to temper the heat, which should roughly equal the natural heat of the human body—the ideal temperature for fermentation. If the degree of heat is too strong, the spirit and subtle parts of the plant will volatilize too quickly, but if the heat is too weak, it will hamper the fermentation process and the substantial parts of the plant will not break up and dissolve.

Next, mix in with the plant matter some brewer's yeast or some flour dissolved in water with bread leaven that has already caused the flour to rise. The vessel should be only half full, however, because the leaven will cause the whole mixture to rise. When the effervescence has passed, allow the leaven to act gently until the crust that forms on the surface begins to subside and precipitate, which usually takes place in two to three days' time in summer or four to five days' time in winter. As soon as this sign appears, quickly transfer the matter to a tinned copper bladder, cover it with a Moor's head, and lute the joints well. Keep the water of the refrigeratory cool in order to condense the vapors. Gradually raise the heat of the fire until the drops begin to follow each other in close succession, then reduce the heat of the fire slowly until the distillate becomes insipid, which will signal the end of operation.

The dose of the spirit is from 6 to 20 drops in a broth; the dose of the volatile salt is from 5 to 20 grains in the plant's own water.[3] These salts are potent antiscorbutics and resolutives, but the spirit and salt of scurvy grass, when prepared in the manner of the nitro-tartarous plants (but, again, without the use of the crucible), is by far the most powerful. This preparation is comparable to Glaser's distillation of watercress described above.

Preparation of Antiscorbutic Water

Wash ½ pound of horseradish roots and cut them into very thin slices. Put them in a large glass cucurbit with 3 pounds of scurvy grass and sea scurvy grass, 1½ pounds of garden cress and watercress, and 1 pound of devil's bit scabious. Pour in 12 pounds of water that has boiled for two hours with a sufficient quantity of cucumber slices and, if available, 4 pounds of Rhine wine. Distill in the bain-marie until nothing further distills.

Pour the water into narrow-necked vials and stop them well. This water serves as an admirable remedy for hematoma and hypochondria. It expels toxins through the sweat and urine, restores the stomach's functions, and strengthens the appetite. Its dose is from 2 to 6 ounces taken in the morning on an empty stomach.[4]

Preparation of Scurvy Grass

Put 4 pounds of horseradish root cut into thin slices in a tinned copper bladder with 6 pounds of garden cress seed, 8 pounds of sea scurvy grass, and 10 pounds of scurvy grass, all finely chopped and crushed. Pour over some good white wine until everything is saturated, then cover the bladder with a Moor's head and lute the joints well. Adapt it to a convenient receiver and set it over the fire to distill the wine. When the spirit becomes weak, it should not be mixed with a previous batch. Continue the fire until the drops become tasteless, then stop the fire.

The dose of the first spirit is from 10 to 40 drops in a white wine. It purifies the blood, eliminates hematomas, and cleanses all the organs. It would be prudent, however, to purge yourself beforehand with the following extract: pass what remains in the bladder through a filter to extract the liquor, then dry and calcine the residue to ashes and extract the salt using the normal method. Evaporate the liquor into a thick syrup and add the salt previously extracted. The dose of the extract is from ½ to 3 drams.[5]

Elecampane Root Extract

The roots of this plant should be pulled in early spring when buds begin to show on the sharp spikes it shoots out of the ground at this time. Gather a large quantity of elecampane roots when the plant is tender and succulent, wash them thoroughly, and cut them into pieces the length of your forefinger. Put them in a cucurbit in the sand bath with a sufficient quantity of clean water. Cover the cucurbit with its alembic head, fit it to a receiver, and lute the joints. Increase the heat gradually until it comes to a boil and the roots are cooked through, then strain and mash the roots to a pulp and preserve them with sugar. This will make an excellent kind of preserve for maladies of the spleen and chest.

But there still remains the saturated spirit of the salt of the plant, which should not go to waste. When the alembic head is invaded by white vapors, this substance will accumulate on the sides. De-lute the alembic head and substitute it for another. Remove the salt with a quill and dissolve it in the spirit already distilled. To make the elecampane extract, use the method already described for other plants. The extract is good for asthma and evacuates thick humors from the stomach, spleen, and bronchi. This preparation may serve as a model for valerian, wild angelica, carline thistle, and contrayerva.[6]

Comfrey Root Extract

Moving on from the aromatic roots, let us now consider those which are insipid and mucilaginous but contain an effective virtue hidden in their viscous juice. This remedy serves as a remarkable cure for hemoptysis. Applied topically, it resolves bruises and fortifies the ligaments and joints after dislocations. Although this extract can be made from common comfrey alone, it is preferable to add the roots, leaves, and flowers of goldenrod, bugle, and common self-heal, as well as the seeds of Saint John's wort, because their balsamic salts will greatly enhance its efficacy.

Take 2 pounds of common comfrey roots, add an equal portion of the roots, leaves, and flowers of the aforementioned species, and wash them thoroughly. Beat them in a mortar and reduce them to a pulp, then add ½ pound of Saint John's wort seeds and crush them in the mortar with a little white wine. Add to the mixture 1 pound of rye breadcrumbs and an equal amount of wheat breadcrumbs, then mix in a little white wine and let it soak to lighten the mixture. Put the mixture in a long-necked matrass, stop it with another inverted matrass, and carefully lute them together. Put them in the bain-marie and digest them slowly until the mixture turns a blood-red color, then allow the furnace to cool, remove the vessels, and strongly express and strain the mixture through a linen filter. Put the expressed liquid in the water bath to make a new digestion—this way the liquor will clarify more easily and leave the useless sediment at the bottom of the vessel. Decant the clear liquid and continue the digestion, periodically separating the clarified liquid. Put the liquor in a cucurbit in the water bath and distill off about two-thirds.

What remains at the bottom is the balsamic extract known as "Blood of Comfrey," which heals internal ulcers, hernias, and wounds. Its dose is from 1 scruple to 1 dram in its own distilled water or in a white wine every day for a minimum of twelve days to a maximum of forty days, or one philosophical month.[7]

Satyrion Root Extract

To obtain the extract of satyrion root, follow the above procedure for the comfrey root extract, only do not combine the satyrion root with any other plants, but add 1 dram of good ambergris per pound of plant matter to be digested.

Its dose is the same as that of the comfrey root extract. This remedy is good for fortifying the womb and increases fertility, hence the plant's name.[8]*

Lady Fern Root Extract

This root should be harvested at the beginning of spring when the lady fern begins to bud and its small yellow shoots emerge from the ground. Wash and clean 40 pounds, cut the roots into pieces, and beat them well in a mortar. Transfer them to a large barrel capable of holding 15 or 20 buckets of water, pour 12 buckets of warm water on the roots and stir well. Fill 2 buckets with rye flour diluted with beer or bread yeast and, when they ferment, add them to the barrel. Stir the mixture well and cover the barrel. Let the mixture ferment for two days, then distill the liquor several times in the copper bladder. When the distillation is complete, rectify the spirit, setting aside the first batch, which is the most efficacious, and so on for the second and third, until it yields nothing more than an insipid phlegm.

This spirit has aperitive and resolutive properties. It opens obstructions of the viscera and especially those of the spleen and the womb. Its dose for the first spirit is from ½ to 2 drams in a vegetable broth (increase the dose by one-third for each subsequent batch).[9]

Colocynth Extract

Reduce some colocynth to a coarse powder and put it in a matrass, then mix in little by little some good distilled vinegar with ½ ounce of Sennert's salt of tartar per pound of vinegar. When the plant matter is well saturated, pour in an additional four fingers of the same vinegar and digest it in the

---

*[The plant name "satyrion," from the Greek σατύριον, is a diminutive of "satyr" (σάτυρος), a class of lecherous woodland deities. —*Trans.*]

ash bath for eight days, shaking and stirring the filled vessel, which should be half full, four times a day. At the end of eight days, strain and percolate the liquor and subject the marc to a new digestion as before. Perform this operation three separate times to get the best of the colocynth, then evaporate the distilled juice to the consistency of an extract.

This anti-scrofulous extract eliminates serosities and cold humors, and calms arthritis. Its dose is from 2 grains to 1 scruple in a Spanish wine.[10]

Elixir of Lemon and Orange Peel

Cut some lemon or orange peels very finely and put 2 ounces in a double circulatory vessel with 1 scruple of ambergris and 6 grains of Levantine musk ground with 2 drams of fine powdered sugar. Pour onto this mixture 8 ounces of the spirit obtained from a distillation of the peels in white wine (this spirit should be very ardent), then stop the vessel and lute the joints. Digest the mixture in the water bath with a slow heat for three days. Allow the vessel to cool, then strain and percolate its contents into a covered vase and preserve the spirit in a well-sealed jar.

These elixirs are powerful cordials that strengthen the heart and overcome syncope. The elixir of orange peel is more effective for women than for men. Their dose is from 1 scruple to 1 dram in their own distilled water.[11]

The Virtue of Plant Liquors

With the exception of the quintessence, the liquor is the best of all possible plant preparations. It is more effective than the water drawn by infusion or by decoction. The previous operations adapted from Glaser in chapter 12 may therefore be esteemed as excellent preparations. These medicaments should be administered in appropriate juleps, herbal teas, or vegetable broths, all of which serve as excellent vehicles. Plant liquors are best preserved when mixed with powdered sugar at a ratio of 4 ounces of powdered sugar per pound of liquor.

The Le Fèvre Method of Preparing Plant Liquors

Nicaise Le Fèvre, who was a faithful disciple of Paracelsus, asserts that the liquor of plants is infinitely more efficacious when it has been obtained by digestion. Here is his general procedure for preparing plant liquors:

Harvest a sufficient quantity of any plant during the *balsamiticum tempus* and beat it in a marble mortar, reducing it to a fine pulp. Put the pulp in a long-necked matrass, so that one-third of the matrass remains empty, and hermetically seal the vessel. Set it to digest in the bain-marie, and heat it with a fire of sawdust for one philosophical month or forty days. At the end of this period, draw out the plant matter, which will have reduced to a liquor, and strain it through a cotton filter, then set it back to digest in the bain-marie to separate the impurities remaining at the bottom of the vessel. Decant the clear liquor or, better, strain it through cotton filter into a glass funnel.

The liquor must be preserved in a vial and combined with its fixed salt, which may be extracted by expression from what remains of the plant. It is best to reduce the *caput mortuum,* that is, the dead earth, feces, or "worthless remains," to ashes and extract the salt by evaporation. When added to the liquor, the salt will both prolong its preservation and enhance its virtue.[12]

The *Primum ens* of Plants

From this liquor it is possible to extract the *primum ens* or "first being" of the plant by purifying it to the highest degree. To do this, put in a matrass equal parts of the liquor of the plant and the water or liquor made from the dissolved salt. Hermetically seal the matrass and expose it to the Sun for forty days. Without any further work the saline water will separate all the heterogeneous and viscous substances that hinder the purity of the noble liquor. At the end of a philosophical month the practitioner will see three distinct separations:

1. The feces or *caput mortuum* of the plant liquor.
2. The plant's *primum ens,* which will be either green and transparent like an emerald or red and clear like an oriental garnet.
3. The saline water imbued with the impure sulfur of the plant.

At this stage, all that remains is to separate the plant's *primum ens,* which requires great care and skill.[13]

The Virtue of the *Primum ens*

Paracelsus, a genial but enigmatic and fanatical man, said concerning the virtue of the *primum ens* that he would have been thought mad had his affirmations not been verified by a number of his disciples. Among these disciples, Nicaise Le Fèvre was certainly one of the most conscientious and clever. He understood a great many of those secrets the spagyric masters merely hinted at, and his works afford ample proof of the value of his teachings.

Here, then, is what Le Fèvre says about the effects of the *primum ens:* "Paracelsus warned practitioners—no doubt to prevent their astonishment—that from the first days of the remedy's use patients would first see their nails fall out, then all the hair of their body, and then they would lose all their teeth, until finally their skin would wrinkle and shrivel and shed like everything else. All these symptoms are outer signs of INNER RENEWAL."[14] Le Fèvre seems to suggest that the panacea penetrates the entirety of the human organism and replenishes it with a new vigor as the external parts, the nails, the hair, the teeth, and the skin, like the excremental byproducts of a commixture or digestion, fall away on their own and without any pain. Paracelsus, moreover, recommends that the practitioner cease to administer the remedy as soon as the patient's skin begins to shed, because, according to Le Fèvre, this "universal sign" indicates that the *action of renewal* has sufficiently spread throughout the body to destroy all the old and impure parts and to resuscitate new ones in their stead. Hence, the "old rind" decays and falls off because it is driven away by new skin forming in its place.

"I know," Le Fèvre adds, "that vulgar scholars and even those who claim to be physicists will regard the virtues I attribute to this remedy as absurd for the simple reason that armchair philosophers, who are incapable of understanding the great arcana of nature, will never be convinced by any proof or experimental demonstration."[15] And so, in order to convince the incredulous, Le Fèvre cites two cases in which the *primum ens melissae* or "first being of lemon balm" produced the very same curious effects. One of Le Fèvre's friends who had absorbed this *primum ens* experienced all of the phenomena described by Paracelsus. But he wished to be fully convinced, and so he tried out the remedy on an old servant woman who was around seventy years of age. He made her take a glass of white wine tinctured with the remedy every morning on an empty stomach. After only twelve days her menstrual cycle, which had long ago expired, returned to her as though she were pubescent in age, and it frightened her to such a degree that her master dared not push the experiment further. But his curiosity got the better of him, and he wanted to know what effect the remedy might have on an animal. So he steeped some seeds in the prepared beverage and fed them to an old hen for eight days. By the sixth day the old hen had lost all her feathers and looked as though she had been plucked, but before the fortnight new feathers had grown back in their place that were more beautiful and colorful than before, and she even began to lay more than her usual number of eggs.

From all this Le Fèvre concludes that disbelievers can easily convince themselves through their own experimentation, provided, however, they are able to understand and carry out the operation according to Paracelsus's instructions.*

---

*It would appear that spagyrists do not often use expression to separate juices from plants, but they are unanimous in claiming that by prior fermentation juices may be obtained whose virtues are more advanced, maturer, and more exalted than the juices obtained by simple expression. However, as we have observed, the juices of certain aqueous or insipid plants will dissipate during the process of fermentation because their principal qualities reside, due to their superficial nature, in their freshness.

15

Introduction to the Spagyric Art

Whoever wishes to verify or supplement what we have written concerning the basic principles of premodern chemistry may easily do so by consulting any number of works on the subject, assuming, however, the reader knows how to ferret out those authors whose knowledge is the most enlightened. As for spagyric chemistry, on the other hand, the masters who discuss its secret principles exercised great caution and reserve and elected to write in an obscure and veiled language that requires of the student not only a natural predisposition toward abstraction, but also some form of initiation, which the student can acquire only by that long and arduous labor which alone is capable of bringing universal laws to light.

Intellectual and intellective intuition is essential to an intimate understanding of the spagyric art. A deep understanding of the arcana cannot be acquired by reason alone, which is limited to the imperfect control of the physical senses. The way of the soul is the only way of election, *for the soul is the divine principle*. Adepts must clear their soul of its instinctive and material gangue *before they can extract soul from matter*. Spagyric distillation is a material analogy for spiritual purification. Spiritual evolution is psychic distillation, and the germ of truth can flower only by the ferment of faith.

Secret Principles of Spagyric Chemistry

The artificial and actual fires described in chapter 12 are the same fires employed in the spagyric art, only in spagyric chemistry the degrees of heat are stabler, subtler, and more precise, the durations more protracted, and the procedures more elaborate. Apart from these artificial fires the masters also speak of other natural and potential fires, which they call "cold fires" because their heat is negative, latent, internal, and inherent in nature. These secret fires, which are not oxidizing but hot and of the nature of Sulfur (the second principle), are also known as "philosophical fires" because they are truly known only by adepts.

The artificial coal fire is actual and unnatural. This fire burns, calcines, sublimates, volatilizes, and desiccates. When tempered by water it becomes a generative, wet, and hot fire of the nature of the element Air in the spring, and it is this fire that is best suited to the operations of nature.

Among the "cold fires," some authors distinguish the following main types:

1. The *oleum vitrioli* or "oil of vitriol" and the *oleum sulphuris* or "oil of sulfur" made by the *campana* or bell-shaped vessel.
2. The essence of common salt and the essence of niter, concentrated by means of the *metallus primus,* which must be dissolved in the spirits, distilled, sublimated, and finally subjected to repeated resolution until the artist obtains a thick and heavy oil with admirable properties.

The latter oil, which we shall discuss in greater detail in chapter 17, fixes and ripens imperfect metals and reduces plants *to their first matter.* Some of the cold fires are so acidic that they will destroy the plant matter, but they are useful in perfecting the mercurial minerals, whereas the permanent and natural fires, which are sulfurous and hot, are well suited to sulfurous minerals and useful for preserving plant seeds in all their strength. *Similia similibus junguntur et dissimilia respuunt:* "Likes attract likes and are repelled by unlikes."

The sulfurous fires have their seat in the oleaginous principle of plants and minerals, but in order to become fires, they must be exalted spagyrically. Almost all fixed salts, and niter especially, can furnish these fires, by which the practitioner may then draw and fix various plant salts. The stinking oil of tartar when distilled and treated spagyrically exceeds all vegetable oils. The fixed salts drawn from the residue by calcination and depuration and treated by spirit of wine yield a powerful and subtle spirit, which we shall also discuss later in greater detail.

The physical base of all mixed bodies is made of Earth and Water. Mercury and Sulfur constitute their generative, evolutive, and vital principle. Salt, the neutral balancing principle, unites the spirit and soul (Mercury and Sulfur) to the material body (Earth and Water). The quintessence or "first being" is the subtlest part of Mercury and Sulfur, united by the volatile Salt and animated by the Celestial Spirit: it is the quintessence that is imbued with the Divine Thought, and it contains virtually within it that form which the spagyric art seeks to extract from mixed bodies.

After the extraction of the quintessence and the separation of the phlegm, there remains at the bottom of the vessel only the *caput mortuum,* the dead earth or feces, which contains the fixed salt. The physical constitution of mixed bodies is therefore made of two essential principles, a median or neutral principle and two passive and material elements. Nevertheless, the elements that engender these principles still manifest in the nature of mixed bodies, and thus some are igneous in nature, others aerial, others aqueous, and others terrestrial, but their qualitative analysis is more rational, for the hot creates Sulfur, the wet creates Mercury, and the dry creates Salt. The cold, as we have said, is an atonic quality that does not give rise to a constituent principle but resides in Earth and Water. Before the spagyric operation on a mixed body may begin, however, practitioners must first determine its elemental nature to know what exactly they can extract from it.

There is also a natural and artificial fire which is the potential cause of the evolution of matter, for every evolutive and generative principle is born of an aerial *warm humidity* of the nature of spring. This fire is made by digging a hole in the earth, filling it with a mixture of chopped hay, straw, and quicklime—in which the sealed vessel containing the plant matter is to be buried—and watering it with warm water. This fire is the *principle of the evolution of matter* by which the sages provoked the animation and involution of atoms to a spiritual latitude. The heat of the Sun is an equally powerful agent of molecular evolution.

The learned Annibal Barlet, whose name is decidedly synonymous with modesty, suggests that the use of cucurbits and the water bath is suitable for plant matter of a "light commixture" and that the ash bath and the sand bath are intended for hard bodies like roots, woods, and seeds. The refrigeratory serves for both soft and hard substances, but it is necessary to macerate them in their own menstruum, if possible, or in a menstruum of the same nature. "In the distillation of *hot herbs*," Barlet says, "the fire must be quick at the beginning, for otherwise the artist will extract nothing but phlegm."[1]

The retort is used for the extraction of waters and oils from woods, seeds, gums, and roots, the matrass (or descent of vapors) for the expression of oils of certain woods such as juniper, guaiac wood, horsetail, and pine as well as some flowers like roses that will change only with difficulty or with a strong fire (*ignis fortis*). Spagyric operations, and distillations in particular, must always begin with an insignificant heat, which should be increased to perfection only gradually. In addition, at the end of these procedures the vessels and their contents must be allowed to cool in a gentle and natural fashion.

The desiccation, trituration, or fermentation of plants whose oils or essences will dissipate easily is not necessary. For such plants—and hot herbs especially, as long as their smell and flavor are still evident—distillation is always preferable. The aromatic essences are only the subtle sulfur and volatile salt of the plant's radical moisture. Any subtle essence or oil is best extracted by the cast-iron cucurbit with its serpentine coil, in an ordinary vehicle and beginning with a boiling fire. Tender and fleshy roots should be distilled like fruits with the alembic in the water or the ash bath, from the minimum to the maximum heat. Ligneous roots, barks, and dry woods should be distilled according to their specific nature either *per descensum* or *per latus* without any vehicle or *per ascensum* in an appropriate menstruum. The hot leaves (whether fresh or dry), flowers, and seeds should also be distilled using the refrigeratory with its serpentine coil, unlike the cold leaves, flowers, and seeds, whose juices must be expressed and then distilled in the bain-marie, whereas other leaves, flowers, and roots require the alembic.

The spagyrists recommend that the plant matter be prepared prior to its distillation and, to this effect, they have recourse to several operations such as fermentation or putrefaction, circulation, and digestion, which differ from each other only slightly.

Fermentation is a reduction of the active and spiritual parts of mixed bodies from potentiality into action, which, in certain cases, must be achieved without the aid of an actual fire, but rather by the potential and natural fire contained within the plant matter itself, which corrupts and divides on its own. Fermentation, in fact, is the key that unlocks the door to an understanding of plant poisons. Through this operation the involute matter and its nature retrograde toward their first form, which is the fermentative and seminal principle.

Circulation is carried out in the circulatory vessel made of two closed cucurbits coupled so that the head of each enters the belly of the other. The ancients also used the pelican or the "vessel of Hermes" for this operation. The plant matter enclosed circulates from below to above by the effect of a gentle and maturing heat and thus saturates itself with its own menstruum. The process of circulation unites the heterogeneous parts and divides the homogeneous ones, forcing the matter to mature in a slow evolution generated by a humid and aerial heat.

Digestion is a slow cooking with a moist and maturing heat that attenuates the matter, divides it, and exalts its active ingredients. This procedure must be performed in a closed vessel.

Now, distillation, as we have said, is the crowning operation of spagyrics, since this is the procedure by which the practitioner extracts the quintessence. The subtle art of spagyric distillation, which has never been known to vulgar distillers, was formerly known only to a few adepts. There are three types of spagyric distillation:

1. Distillation *per ascensum,* where the fire is placed below the vessel to make the spirits ascend, is the most common method and is particularly suitable for distillations of spirituous and volatile substances.

2. Distillation *per latus,* where the apparatus is so arranged that the spirits pass horizontally, is performed with the retort and is particularly well suited to dense materials that contain heavy oils and require a stronger fire.

3. Distillation *per descensum,* where the fire is placed above the vessel to flush out the spirits from below, is capable of detaching the most tenacious components from plants, for which reason the ancient chemists held it in especially high regard.

The most essential apparatus for distillation is the alembic. The structure of this instrument varies according to the quantity, substance, species, nature, and consistency of the plant matter to be distilled. The ancients mention seven types of alembics:

1. The *earthenware alembic,* little used due to its precarious nature.
2. The *glass alembic,* used for an anodyne heat.
3. The *bain-marie,* the most commonly used.
4. The *serpentine alembic,* by far the most famous.
5. The *spirit boiler,* used for large quantities of plant matter.
6. The *retort,* used for strong fires.
7. The *circulatory vessel* made of two cucurbits, used for rectifications.

Finally, it is fitting for any modern student of spagyrics to consider what factors guided the masters in their use of these various stills, because there is every reason to believe that the shapes of these vessels derived from a theoretical framework that was markedly different from the one our chemists have today. We shall do our utmost in what follows to penetrate the intimate nature of spagyric operations according to the conceptions of the masters of the art, but the bulk of our efforts will be directed toward understanding the subtle art of spagyric distillation, because this is the operation by which matter exhales its soul. Before doing so, however, it would be prudent to provide a brief summary of the classifications of spagyric chemical operations.

The spagyric art consists of five general chemical operations: digestion, distillation, sublimation, calcination, and coagulation.

1. *Digestion* is subdivided into nine secondary operations: depuration, infusion, maceration, insolation, dissolution, fusion, fermentation, putrefaction, and circulation.
2. *Distillation* has five subdivisions: rectification, cohobation, filtration, decantation, and deliquium or deliquescence.
3. *Sublimation* consists of only two secondary operations: dry and adherent elevation and separation.
4. *Calcination* includes twelve subdivisions or varieties: dephlegmation, decrepitation, evaporation, ignition, incineration, precipitation, fumigation, reverberation, stratification, cementation, amalgamation, and revivification.
5. *Coagulation* has four subdivisions: digestion, congelation, vitrification, and fixation.

The reader may find detailed descriptions of each of these primary and secondary operations in the works of Christophe Glaser, Antoine Baumé, and Nicolas de Locques. We would not recommend the writings of Nicolas Lémery, however, since he is far too close-minded on the subject of spagyrics.

General and Specific Rules of the Spagyric Art

◢ **Spagyric calcination** is the transformation of matter into another form by increasing, rather than decreasing and destroying, its radical moisture, which separates its impurities and disposes the body to shed its seed.

◢ **Spagyric sublimation** ennobles and exalts the nature of mixed bodies and volatilizes their spirits in a closed vessel so that they fall back onto the matter, which they dissolve, elevate, and subtilize.

◢ **Spagyric dissolution** breaks down matter through a process of humid corruption by attenuating its dry parts or by subtilizing its aqueous parts, thus separating the pure from the impure.

◢ **Spagyric putrefaction** is the secret of the art. It is either simple or double, natural or against nature. In the first case, the outer form is destroyed and the essential nature preserved. In the second case, the substance of the mixed body is reincruded back to its original form or first vegetable nature, after which it is impossible to restore it to its previous form.

- **Spagyric coagulation** is an important operation, but it differs from the vulgar procedure only insofar as the coagulator is known exclusively to masters of the art.
- **Spagyric distillation** is natural or artificial. In the natural method, the cold is the only agent that fixes or condenses and the Sun the only fire that volatilizes or rarefies the moisture, and not from without but *from within,* which descends anew as dew. Artificial distillation is analogous to spagyric sublimation.

Patience is required in this art, for the longer the plant matter is subjected to a maturing digestion via *warm moisture,* the more it evolves and the better it lends itself to distillation. Maximum evolution can be achieved by digesting the matter in the water bath or the steam bath for two months prior to the first distillation, for one month prior to the second distillation, for three weeks before the third distillation, for a fortnight before the fourth distillation, for eight days before the fifth distillation, for four days before the sixth distillation, and for two days before the seventh distillation. In addition, each distillation must be regulated according to a specific heat regimen.

To extract the quintessence from a plant, it must be distilled seven or ten times *at least:*

1. The first distillation begins in the first degree of the *water bath,* increases gradually to the second degree, then to the third degree, then decreases gradually back down to the first degree.
2. The second distillation is similar to the first.
3. The third distillation begins in the first degree of the *ash bath,* increases slowly to the third degree, and descends back to the first degree.
4. The fourth distillation is analogous to the third.
5. The fifth distillation begins in the first degree of the *sand bath,* then increases to the second and third degrees, and descends slowly back to the first degree.
6. The sixth distillation begins the process of decreasing the type

of fire. It returns to the *ash bath* and proceeds like the third distillation.

7. The seventh distillation or rectification begins in the first degree of the *water bath* and rises slowly up to the third degree, remaining there until the operation's conclusion.

Thus, each distillation individually consists in increasing and decreasing the degrees of the fires, and all seven distillations as a whole consist in increasing and decreasing the fires themselves. These operations require a great deal of knowledge, skill, and experience. Moreover, the spagyrist must be vigilant with respect to the degrees of heat, which must never be exceeded.*

Circulatory Vessels

The shape of the circulatory vessels is of great importance. The preferred vessels for circulations are of two types:

1. The "double vessel," which is a circulatory vessel made from two twin vessels having a shape of a gourd by connecting them to each other with the beaks starting from the head of each vessel and sloping downward into the belly of the other—these crossed beaks form the shape of an X, and a *pertuis* or small aperture sits atop each vessel for introducing materials.

2. The pelican or "circulatory of Hermes," which is a tall earthenware cucurbit, the head of which connects to the belly by two hollow handles through which the waters and spirits circulate.

The heat required for circulations can be attained in several ways, as described below.

Differences between Circulation and Digestion

Each of these operations requires a specific type of vessel. For digestions, the plant matter, which is often coarse and abundant, should be

---

*Isidore of Seville says that for the ash bath, juniper wood is the best and the most stable wood (*Etymologies*, 17.7.35 [ed. Lindsay]).

placed in spacious vessels that are broad on the top but fashioned in such a manner that one can adapt a blind alembic without a beak, so that when the matter is digested, the residue may be drawn out once the blind alembic is removed. The blind alembic is then replaced with a beak alembic, but if the matter is clear and has separated from its *caput mortuum,* it must be transferred to the circulatory cucurbit described above with two hollow ducts in the form of handles connecting the head to the belly. The pelican, which Pseudo-Llull, Philipp Ulstad, and many others consider to be the noblest circulatory vessel, is used for the circulation of waters, spirits, or liquors. The main difference between digestion or fermentation and circulation, then, is that whereas digestion is suitable for coarse and undeveloped raw materials and requires a broad cucurbit and blind alembic, circulation is necessary for liquid, oily, or subtle materials and requires a circulatory vessel.

To attain a putrefactive heat, dig a pit in the earth, lay down a bed of pulverized quicklime about four fingers' thick, and cover the quicklime with a bed of straw or hay about two and a half feet thick. Bury the vessel in the straw or hay and water the whole pit with warm water to ferment the lime. The top of the vessel should extend above the bed of straw or hay so that it is exposed to the air, and the bed of straw or hay must be rewatered with warm water once a week. It suffices to pour more water over the matter once the first water is absorbed, and the lime must be changed when ebullition is no longer possible.

If this fire is not a viable option, the practitioner must resort to the bain-marie. But this bath must maintain a continuous heat, otherwise the virtue of the plant matter will spoil. When the fire is regulated at a constant temperature, the best part of the plant will float over the feces after a short amount of time, and it will work continuously to clarify, purify, and exalt itself. The matter to be digested should be enclosed in long-necked glass matrasses that are very smooth and filled only two-thirds full.

Digestions can also be performed using the heat of the Sun during a heat wave. Place the matrasses in thick earthenware vessels filled with water and expose them to the Sun, using metallic mirrors, if necessary, to reflect the Sun's rays onto the vessels. Another type of digestion can be made in October in the marc of grapes during their fermentation; this heat is soft and natural and causes a slow and maturing digestion. Some authors recommend separating the plant juice or oil after the initial digestion and then setting them to redigest or circulate prior to distillation.

Paracelsus, however, recommends that the plant matter be reduced to a pulp and placed in closed vessels in the steam bath for forty days, after which time the liquor is to be poured out and filtered and the fixed salt, once extracted from the residue by calcination and depuration, dissolved therein. The liquor and its salt must then be enclosed in a well-luted vessel and exposed to the Sun or digested in the water bath for another forty days. All that remains, then, is to distill according to the art. This secret operation is an excellent method of plant preparation, but Paracelsus concealed in his works other and even more secret operations, the mysteries of which we attempt to unveil in this book.

The Seal of Hermes

Most often the noble spirit or sulfur requires a Hermetic enclosure so that its subtle virtue is not exhaled by exaltation of the fire. In such cases the practitioner must resort to the most noble of sigillations known as the "seal of Hermes." To make this seal, clog the top of the long neck of the matrass with clay after filling approximately one-third of its volume with the material to be digested. Tilt the long neck toward the opening of the lit furnace until the glass reddens from the violence of the fire. Take strong flat pincers, the end of which will redden in the fire, and gently grasp the top of the neck of the matrass to warm it still further, then tighten the pincers to close up the neck: turn the pincers slowly, twisting the glass in a single turn.

The vessel should never be placed into a bath until the neck has cooled down, for otherwise it will break. To open the vessel after the operation, wrap the top of the neck several times around with a thick cotton thread soaked in spirit of wine or coated with sulfur and set it over the flame. Once the glass becomes hot, simply wipe the area with a damp cloth and the collar will break clean off.

The Use of Potential and Sulfurous
Fires in Cultivation

Operations of spagyric horticulture are usually performed on seeds. Infuse some seeds in a liquid composed of fifteen parts filtered rainwater to one part fire, potential or sulfurous, dissolved in rainwater. Infuse the seeds until they become soft and are about to putrefy. These seeds once planted will grow more quickly and vigorously than uninfused seeds of the same plant species, and their fruits will be more fleshy and ripe.

The Paracelsian Method of Extracting
the Quintessence from Plants

Pile and chop the chosen plant and let it putrefy in the steam bath for thirty or forty days. Express the juice and distill it in the water bath. Return the distilled liquor to its feces and let it putrefy for eight days, then distill it several more times and as the colors change the quintessence will ascend through the alembic and the body will remain at the bottom of the vessel along with a portion of its essential water. Pour all of the quintessence back onto the body and let it putrefy once more for four days. Distill as before and return the liquor to its residue. Let it digest in the pelican for six days, after which time it will turn into a thick liquor, then distill it in the water bath. The aqueous body will separate, and the quintessence will remain at the bottom. Separate the quintessence from the impure juices and digest it once more so that it deposits its feces. All that remains, then, is to rectify it one last time, and the quintessence will be imbued with the exalted virtues of the plant.[2]

The Pseudo-Llullian Method of Extracting
the Quintessence from Plants

Pile and chop the chosen plant and put it in a closed vessel with true quintessence of wine and expose it to the spring Sun or put it in the steam bath for three days. Next, begin the distillation with a slow heat so that the drops appear gradually. Return the liquor to its feces, digest it for two days, and then distill it two times. Pour the spirit back over its body once more and digest it for one full day, then distill it three times and rectify the spirit. It is important to note, however, that the quintessence of wine added at the beginning of this operation should equal only one-third the amount of plant matter.[3]

The Ulstad Method of Extracting the Quintessence from Plants

Chop the desired parts of the chosen plants and pound them in a mortar with a tenth part of cleaned common salt, then set them in the circulatory to ferment in the steam bath for thirty or forty days. Next, distill them with the beak alembic in the water bath, gradually increasing the heat to the third degree. Set the distilled water aside, then draw out the residue and pulverize it in the marble mortar. Put the residue in a well-luted blind alembic with the distilled water, and distill them in the bain-marie, gradually increasing the heat to the second degree. Repeat these operations three times: pound, soak, mix, digest, and distill, always decreasing the fire to the first degree at the end of each operation. The second digestion should last twenty-one days; the third, fourteen days; and the fourth, eight days. After the fourth and perfect distillation, put everything in the circulatory in a steam bath of the first degree—or use the heat of the summer Sun or the marc of grapes—for one month or forty days, then distill once more with the beak alembic in the water bath.

Afterward, calcine the feces and draw out the salt by depuration. Dissolve the salt in the liquor and let them circulate together for seven days, then distill the spirit three times separately until it is pure and rectified.[4] Any salt remaining after the final rectification must be separated and discarded.

This operation will render the true quintessences of seeds, leaves, and roots. The practitioner may follow this operative procedure to prepare the majority of simples.*

---

*Mountain arnica, which was poorly known among the ancients, contains a quintessence whose virtues cannot be ascribed to any other plant. This quintessence resides chiefly in its flowers. We recommend preparations of this plant, whose nature takes after wormwood, lemon balm, and saffron, to adepts in particular.

The Le Fèvre Method of Extracting the Quintessence from Plants

Grind the chosen plant in a marble mortar and reduce it to a pulp, then put it in a long-necked matrass sealed with the seal of Hermes, and set it to digest in the steam bath for forty days. At the end of the philosophical month, open the matrass and extract all of the plant matter, separating the liquid part by passing it through a cloth filter. Put it in the bain-marie for a full day, then decant or filter through a cotton filter using a funnel.

Draw the fixed salt from the residue in the manner of the art and dissolve it in the liquor, then put the mixture in a hermetically sealed matrass and expose it to the Sun or a fire of lime and straw for six weeks. At the end of this period, you will see the plant's *primum ens* floating on the surface, which will be colored either green and transparent or red and clear depending on the nature of the Salt, Sulfur, and Mercury that constitute the plant.[5] Finally, separate the liquid "first being" and distill it in the spagyric manner.

The Time Required for Philosophical Distillation

Whoever knows nature in all its movements must operate in non-imitation in the required time frames. Make a steam bath so that the water boils and the containing vessel is surrounded by water vapors. The distillation will commence if you have previously heated the plant matter by the heat of water and you can slowly count to *seven* between each drop that falls into the receiver. According to Franz de le Boë (alias Franciscus Sylvius), this is the only true philosophical distillation.[6]

Spagyric Distillation of Wine

Take a very good natural wine, neither too young nor too old, but generous, in any quantity and set it in the vessel to distill with the alembic positioned so that its beak enters the upper part of the receiver. Lute the joints well with a mixture of flour and egg whites brought to the consistency of honey and, as Pseudo-Llull recommends, with a mind inclined toward sapience.[7]

Set the container on the tripod of arcana, which is a circular iron tray pierced with seven round holes and supported by three very short feet, then place the tripod on a bain-marie equipped with a large boiler sealed to the wall and half filled with water. It may then be placed in the *furnus acediae* or "furnace of sloth," which the practitioner must never move.

Begin with a slow fire (*ignis lentus*) under the spirit boiler until the water is lukewarm, increase the heat slowly until it reaches the first degree of heat, and maintain this temperature for a lengthy period of time. Increase the heat imperceptibly to the second degree, then to the third, and slowly descend back down to the first degree. After the completion of this procedure the practitioner may distill in the manner of the art by returning the liquor obtained to its feces, without washing the vessel.

Putrefaction of Wine by Circulation

To obtain the quintessence of very pure and evolved wine, the practitioner may employ several means prior to distillation. First digest the crushed grapes in their own water for a fortnight, then filter this water after adding the tartar extracted from the marc by calcination and depuration. All that remains, then, is to circulate this liquor in the circulatory for four days before subjecting it to distillation.

If the wine is already prepared, however, circulate it in one of the appropriate vessels for seven days, then filter and return it to the circulatory for six days, then filter again and recirculate for five days, and so on and so on, decreasing the duration each circulation by one day and filtering the liquor between each circulation, making seven circulations in all.

Circular Distillation of Wine

Once the digested wine is ready for distillation, pour it into one of the noble vessels which the masters describe as suitable for the best circulations. Immerse it in a large vessel two-thirds full of water and expose it to the sweltering Sun. It may also be placed in the water bath at the first degree or a little higher, depending on whether the plant matter is more or less tempered or subtilized from the previous digestion.

Circulate the digested wine for a lengthy period of time, until the quintessence manifests, which you will recognize by the smooth, sweet, warm, penetrating, and subtle flavor of the liquor. If at the bottom of the vessel there should remain a murky and liquid residue like a whitish cloud, separate it from the liquor by distillation, then recirculate it in a clean vessel, leaving the thick residue in the first. The more the liquor circulates at a slow heat, the more ennobled and exalted it will become, as it will attract more celestial influences, to the benefit of whoever partakes of it.

A Simple Method of Extracting the Quintessence from Wine

Take a certain quantity of very good red or white wine, a little sweet to the taste, and distill it through the alembic, four times, while closely monitoring the degrees of heat. Next, put this spirit in the pelican with two handles, lute the *pertuis* or small aperture that sits atop the vessel so that the spirits cannot escape, and circulate it according to the art. Matter purified by frequent circulatory distillations and by repeated sublimations becomes increasingly noble. From elemental matter is made non-elemental matter, an incorruptible body in the image of heaven, from which it draws its virtue.

When the liquor is sufficiently sublimated in the distillatory, open the *pertuis* at the top of the pelican. If the matter is pure, a sweet aroma will rise to delight the senses of practitioners and incense their entire home with a heavenly fragrance. But if the odor is bland, impure, and raw, then the lid of the *pertuis* must be reluted and the circulatory distillation continued for as long as necessary or, as Pseudo-Llull says, "until the liquor appears in the form of vegetable Mercury, whose sweet smell and sweet taste are signs of its perfection."[8]

Extracting the Quintessence from Wine without Fire

Put the first spirit of wine in a long-necked and well-luted matrass and bury the matrass in a pit filled with chopped straw and quicklime. Water everything with warm water, as we have instructed previously. This can be done in another manner by placing the matrass in a barrel two-thirds full of tepid water and burying it in the marc of grapes while it ferments. After forty days, transfer the spirit to the two-handled circulatory of Hermes and expose it to the heat of the Sun for seven days.

Exalting the Power of a Spirit of Wine

Grind in a mortar 1 ounce of sugar candy (per half gallon of wine) and add a tenth of an ounce of fine flowers of sulfur (*flores sulphuris*).* Put this powder in a cooking pot with a little wine, cover, and cook slowly for a long period of time. Combine this solution with the wine to be distilled and operate according to the rules of spagyric distillation. The spirit obtained will be much more ardent than if one were to extract it without this prior preparation.

Spirit of Essential Wine of the Adepts

Digest any quantity of wine for a fortnight in the water bath. Distill the spirit and rectify it three times to remove the phlegm. Mix 2 pounds of this spirit with 6 pounds of the same wine, then distill, removing only 2 pounds of spirit. Mix these 2 pounds of spirit with another 6 pounds of digested wine, and distill off 2 more pounds of spirit. Repeat these operations seven times until you obtain the true sulfur of the wine, which should be so volatile that when poured out in drops it evaporates before hitting the ground.

Pseudo-Llull's *Aquae vitae*

1st Aqua vitae: Take equal parts fennel root, butcher's broom, maidenhair fern, asparagus, horseradish, parsley, eryngo, common gromwell, and endive, grind them in a mortar and mix them together, then put them in a cucurbit with alcohol or spirit of wine. Distill seven times according to the rules of the spagyric art. This water breaks up and dissolves kidney and bladder stones.

---

*[Flowers of sulfur (*flores sulphuris*) is a very fine, bright yellow sulfur powder produced by sublimation and deposition; see, e.g., John Quincy, *Pharmacopoeia officinalis & extemporanea,* 2nd ed., 316. —*Trans.*]

2nd Aqua vitae: Take equal parts clove, nutmeg, mastic, leopard's-bane, zedoary, galangal, long pepper, lemon peel, sage, old man's beard or marjoram, dill, nard, aloeswood, cubeb pepper, cardamom, lavender, mint, pennyroyal, oregano, sweet flag, germander, musk, and yellow bugle, grind them in a mortar and mix them together, and let them ferment in spirit of wine for three days prior to spagyric distillation. The virtues of this water are similar to those of the aromatic liquors, but much more effective.

3rd Aqua vitae: Take equal parts spurge, sagapenum, opopanax, pyrethrum, caper, bdellium, long pepper, cubeb pepper, castor oil, and zedoary, add a little ambergris, grind them in a mortar and mix them together, then ferment and distill according to the rules of the spagyric art. The virtues of this water are marvelous and manifold.[9]

Aqua vitae for All Infirmities and Early Onset of Old Age

Mix 4 pounds of rectified *aqua vitae* with 4 drams each of cinnamon, white ginger, and nutmeg; 4 ounces of peppermint and cinnamon bark; 2 ounces of thyme and wild thyme; 4 ounces of honey; and 2 ounces of pure flowers of sulfur. Let the mixture putrefy in a glass vessel for fourteen days, then circulate the liquor in the circulatory vessel for three days. Afterward, distill with the alembic in the water bath three times and you will obtain a very pure and salutary water whose virtues are extraordinary.

Since all preparations of *aquae vitae* are very similar, it is easy for practitioners to compose various panaceas for all diseases or to tailor-make them to treat special cases. First consult the classifications of medicinal plants in chapter 2 and select several plants having the same nature in order to form a group of plants targeted to a specific illness. Next, prepare the *aqua vitae* in accordance with the directives prescribed in the preceding formulae. By adhering to these directives the practitioner can compose an admirable *aqua vitae* for paralysis, epilepsy, and all contagious diseases using the following ingredients: ½ pound each of sage, oregano, hyssop, savory, salad burnet root, valerian root, and wormwood; 2 drams each of rue, bistort root, and parsley root; 4 drams of sugar of roses (*saccharum rosaceum*);* ½ dram of herb bennett, polypody, and tormentil; ½ ounce of rosemary, parsley, chervil, lavender, and marjoram; 2 ounces of red and white roses; and 4 drams of juniper berries. This formula is only *exempli gratia*. In fact, the practitioner can make excellent *aquae vitae* using only one, two, or three plant ingredients.

Stomachic and Compensatory
Aqua vitae

Mix 4 liters of pure *aqua vitae* with 4 liters of Malvasia wine. Add to this mixture 3 ounces of cinnamon, 1 ounce of cloves, 1½ ounces of white ginger, 1½ ounces of Indian neem, 2 drams of galangal, 1 ounce of nutmeg, ½ ounce of mace, ½ ounce of cubeb pepper and hyssop, 1 ounce of herb bennett, and 1½ ounces of white roses. Crush the mixture and transfer it to a large cucurbit that can hold sixteen pounds of liquid. Add 3 ounces of white sugar, 6 ounces of raisins and figs, and ½ ounce of camphor. Carefully lute the cucurbit and set it in the Sun for twenty days, ten days before Nativity of Saint John the Baptist (June 24th) and ten days after. Afterward, pour out the water, distill it three times through the alembic, and store it in a dry place.

Its dose is ½ teaspoon taken on an empty stomach.[10]

Purifying, Vivifying, and Comforting
Aqua vitae

Pound in a marble mortar and then mix together 12 ounces of sage; 4 drams each of nutmeg, cloves, white ginger, grains of paradise, and cinnamon; 1 ounce of laurel oil; 1 dram of fresh castor oil; ½ dram of spikenard and rosemary; 1 ounce of rue leaves; 2 drams of marjoram leaves; and 2 drams of lemon peel. All of these ingredients should be

---

*[The remedy known as *saccharum rosatum* or "sugar of roses" is prepared in the following manner: "Take of red rose leaves, the whites being cut off, and speedily dried in the sun an ounce, white sugar a pound, melt the sugar in rose-water and juice of roses of each two ounces which being consumed by degrees, put in the rose leaves in powder, mix them, put it upon a marble, and make it into lozenges according to art" (Nicholas Culpeper, *The Complete Herbal*, 316–17). —*Trans*.]

fresh. If it is not possible to use fresh ingredients, then powderize them and let them saturate in a good white wine. Digest the mixture in the water bath for one month, then distill with the alembic in the water bath. Return the liquor to its residue and redistill, then distill in the ash bath for the third and final time and preserve the liquor in a sealed vessel.[11]

This liquor is not suitable for hot or choleric temperaments, but it can cure all phlegmatic and lymphatic diseases, both internal and external, and can even restore one's youth. A similar and much simpler liquor can be made with 4 pounds of ordinary *aqua vitae* and 1 ounce each of rosemary, cloves, and white ginger.

Fortifying and Soothing *Aqua vitae*

Roughly grind together equal parts of white ginger, cinnamon, cubeb pepper, clove, nutmeg, mace, cardamom, Indian neem, galangal, and long pepper. Pour six parts of pure *aqua vitae* over the spices, put the mixture in a cucurbit, digest with the blind alembic for fourteen days, then distill in the water bath with a very slow fire. Return the spirit to the plant matter and redistill for eight days. Do this three times. Next, reduce to a coarse powder 3 drams each of sage leaves, rue leaves, fresh castor oil, lemon peel, laurel seeds, lavender, and rosemary flowers. Mix them with *aqua vitae,* then digest, distill, and prepare them in the manner of the example below concerning the quintessence of aromatic plants. After this preparation, unite the two spirits and distill them three times together and you will obtain a beneficial *aqua vitae* that is useful against phlegmatic diseases.

This liquor should be taken in the morning at a dose of 2 drams in a good white wine. It will not only strengthen the weak, but also rejuvenate the complexion.

Equilibrating *Aqua vitae*

Combine *aqua vitae,* distilled several times, rosemary, cinnamon, clove, ginger, and mace with 1 ounce of fine flowers of sulfur. Circulate the mixture for three days, then filter it carefully and distill it four times.

This equilibrating water, when taken in a small dose once in the morning and once in the evening, protects against infectious diseases.

The Most Virtuous *Aqua vitae*

Pound and mix together 1 ounce each of fresh sage (with flowers), rosemary, white ginger, cloves, nutmeg, grains of paradise, galangal, sweet flag, and zedoary; ½ ounce of eastern pellitory-of-the-wall seed; 2 drams each of mace, cubeb pepper, rue leaves, lavender, marjoram, and red roses; 1½ drams each of Mithridate and "Venice Treacle";* 1½ drams each of laurel oil, borage flowers, bugloss, lemon peel, rosemary flowers, angelica, rhapontic rhubarb, common centaury, mint, apple mint, and feverfew; ½ dram each of fresh castor oil, vervain (with flowers), betony, aloeswood, opobalsam, carpobalsam, spike lavender, acorn, and peony seeds; and ½ dram each of basil seed, fennel seed, anise seed, speedwell, and saffron. Combine these ingredients with 10 pounds of distilled spirits and digest for four full days. Then distill three more times, each time returning the distilled liquor to its feces. Make a paste with 2 pounds of fine honey, 1 dram of camphor, and 2 ounces of flowers of sulfur and circulate it for ten days with the liquor. On the eleventh day, separate the liquor from the *caput mortuum* and rectify it three times in the alembic.[12]

The virtues of this *aqua vitae* are so numerous we cannot extol one above the others.

The Croll Method of Preparing Herb Salts

Gather the following in equal parts: leaves and roots of black hellebore, blessed thistle, and garden angelica; roots of parsley, angelica, centaury,

---

*[Mithridate (*mithridatium, mithridaticum,* or *mithridatum*) is a semimythical drug allegedly created by Mithridatus IV in the first century BCE. The theriac of Andromachus (*theriaca Andromachi*) or "Venice Treacle," as it was later known among English apothecaries, is a first-century CE variation on Mithridate created by Andromachus the Elder, physician to Emperor Nero. Both Mithridate and "Venice Treacle" were extremely complex and highly sought-after remedies, each consisting of over sixty ingredients. See especially the monograph by the German alchemist Andreas Libavius, *De theriaca Andromachi senioris, ex Mithridatio nata, & a temporibus Neronis Principis in Imperio Romano per Graecos & Lationos Medicos celebrata. —Trans.*]

salad burnet, tormentil, and celandine; leaves and flowers of chicory; and leaves of Saint John's wort, arum, great mullein, vincetoxicum, and cinquefoil.

First dry all these herbs in the shade *away from the heat of the Sun,* then chop them up, put them in a small barrel, and saturate them with a decoction of hops and ferment. Place the barrel in a hothouse and stir the mixture from time to time, so that it swells. This process should last three weeks, and the barrel should be kept covered. Distill everything through the copper retort, refreshing the spirits as in distillations of *aqua vitae.* Moderately rectify the distilled spirit, reduce the residue of the herbs to ashes, and draw the salt by depuration. After drying, dissolve the salt in its spirit. Distill the spirit in the water bath, pour it back over the salt, and repeat until nothing more can be extracted. Mix the extracts and digest them in the water bath for four days, then separate the spirit from the feces by filtering it through a brown paper filter. Distill these extracts in a boiling water bath and the salt will ascend together with the spirit. Cohobate once more and distill the spirit in the sand bath, then mix it with its phlegm and let them stand in a cool place while the salt precipitates. Separate this subtle salt—which, according to Paracelsus, possesses countless virtues—and save the spirit for other extractions.

This salt is good for all diseases that require evacuation and for all putrefactions, obstructions, and superfluous humidities. Administer it with essence of saffron, wormwood, Malvasia wine, or herbal juices. Its dose is from 2 to 20 grains, depending on the patient's age.[13]

The Cold Quintessence

All fermentation degenerates into spirit or alcohol, and almost all quintessences are hot in nature. Yet Conrad Gessner, otherwise known as the "Swiss Pliny," gives a formula for a cold quintessence whose nature is contrary to that of the *aquae vitae.* Here is its preparation:

Gather 1 pound each of old man's beard flowers and coltsfoot flowers that grow on the water and have broad leaves and yellow flowers (this is most likely a reference to the water lily), ½ pound each of lettuce seed and water purslane seed, and 2 scruples of black nightshade flowers, all in their greenness. Distill these plants seven times and put the water in a glass matrass. Bury the matrass deep in the earth and leave it there for several days. After using it, store it in a deep and cool place.[14]

This liquor arrests menstruation, interrupts perspiration, incites the appetite, calms migraines, and cures cankers. In short, it destroys any disease that is hot in nature such as inflammation of the eyes, sexual excitation, fistulas, and heartburn. It may be taken at a dose of 1 teaspoon in the morning or evening or by injection or enema.*

Quintessence of the Four Elements

Distill an excellent red wine three times in the water bath, surrounding the alembic or receiver with *tepid* water to temper the heat during the beginning of the distillation. Next, remove this lukewarm water and replace it with cold water. The vessel containing this water must be at least one palm's width and made of red tinned copper. It should also have a *pertuis* set in the middle that is similar to the one on the distillatory so that they may be luted together with precision. When the wine is well distilled and you can no longer draw anything from it, pour it back into the distillatory through the *pertuis* on top and lute it immediately and with great care.

Distill the new wine and set apart the phlegm, of which we shall speak in due course. Next, put the distilled wine in the furnace of sloth, in the sand bath called *acedia*. Lacking this furnace, make use of the steam bath, but arrange it in such a manner that the water vapor circulates around the vessel to bathe the distilled wine with a continual, sweet, and digestive warmth. To be certain that all of the spirit has distilled, check to see that there are no more drops coming out of the alembic, which is a sure sign that there is no more spirit in the matter. After having set the spirit aside, immediately fill the cucurbit with *aqua*

---

*Pseudo-Llull gives the following formula to obtain a water contrary to the nature of *aquae vitae:* white camphor, rose, white and black pepper, chicory, water purslane, violet, marsh mallow root, black nightshade, maidenhair fern, houseleek, white stonecrop, hog's fennel seed, and golden thistle. See "Ars operativa medica," in *Ioannis de Rvpescissa qvi ante CCCXX. annos vixit,* 182.

vitae, then place the alembic above it and carefully lute them together. Next, distill in the ash or water bath using the acedious furnace.

The distillation should be performed in the following manner: after each distillation, reunite the phlegm remaining in the distillatory with the first spirit to ripen and improve the new spirit of each distillation. This should be done seven or nine times, so that the quintessence draws and separates in very small quantities. Sixty measures of wine should render one glassful of essential liquor, which, if it is not quickly and properly sealed, will volatilize with extreme rapidity. Great care must be taken when drawing it from the container so that it does not evaporate.

The four elements are separated in the following manner: mix all of the waters drawn from the previous distillations and pour them into the caldarium (warming vessel) of the aforementioned furnace or into a large cucurbit. Distill them in the water bath to extract all of the phlegm until nothing else distills. Upon removing the receptacle you will find in the cucurbit a dark matter like molten pitch. But to obtain this dark matter in a quicker fashion, evaporate a portion of the phlegm in an iron vessel over a coal fire until the residue thickens to a tender pitch, then transfer it to the cucurbit. Pour more phlegm into the iron vessel and, after it thickens and evaporates, add the dark matter to the quantity in the cucurbit. Repeat this process until all the phlegm has evaporated.

Dry the dark matter over a slow fire, then add the quintessence already extracted, but do so with extreme caution so that the quintessence does not volatilize: soak the matter thoroughly and see that the two are well combined. Set them to digest in the bain-marie, then distill them through the alembic. Pour the distillation water over the black sludge and feces and distill again, then rejoin the water and the feces, digest them together once more, and distill the water. This process must be repeated several times. The seventh distillation will render the medicinal liquor called *Sanguis humanus* or "Human Blood," to which the alchemists attribute the element Air, and so the practitioner will now have two elements: Air and Water.

Continue by distilling through the alembic the oil that remains in the thick residue or dark matter at the bottom of the distillatory in the ash bath and keep this oil separate. The dry black earth that remains in the cucurbit can refine the quintessence by its ferment. Distill the dark matter with all of the quintessence until they are well combined. When drops begin to emerge that resemble a clear oil, remove the receptacle and substitute it for another, larger one—because of the strength of the spirits—and set it over a median fire for twenty-four hours, for a more violent fire will cause the earth to rise. Once the oily spirit has passed, increase the fire until nothing else distills. Its earth, remaining dry, will have the smell of something burning. Mix it with the phlegm of the *aqua vitae* so that there is four times more water than earth and transfer them to a glass vessel or a lead-sealed earthenware vessel. When the earth has settled and the water has evaporated from the heat of the bath, add the same amount of water as before and repeat this procedure until the earth becomes inodorous. Now that the earth is well cleared of its water, combine it with the quintessence once more and slowly distill the liquor.

Rectify the liquor in the following manner: combine the Earth in the form of a dry and fine powder with the two elements previously obtained, namely Water and Air. Circulate them in the water bath for three days and three nights. Then distill this ardent water, which is pure Fire, so that three elements are exalted in the quintessence. Calcine the remaining earth to a whitish ash in the reverberatory furnace. Prior to this, however, the earth must be put in two well-luted terrines and set in a bed of quicklime for twelve days in order to prepare it for reverberation. After complete calcination, mix it with the spirit of the Fire element already obtained and circulate them in the water bath for three days and three nights. Then distill seven times, and calcine the earth by reverberation an equal number of times. When the earth no longer dissolves in the spirit, it is then evolved and ready for use, for this is the Stone of the Philosophers, and not the Salt, as some say.

Each of the four elements appear in this divine operation: the phlegm is the element Water; the oil is the element Air; the rectified spirit is the element Fire; and the evolved earth is the element Earth. This forms the basis of the work by which gold is solved and made ready to render its seed and transmutate into a universal medicine. The practitioner, however, must be careful not to make use of the liquor of Fire, the last to exit, because its heat is such that if taken internally, it would dry out the blood and the organs, but it is safe to use when it has been united with its Earth to make medicine from gold.

Preparation of Subtle Earth with *Aqua vitae*

Make *aqua vitae* from wine, rectify it three or four times so that it is deprived of all moisture, then separate the earth from its phlegm. Put the phlegm in a caldarium and cook it until it reaches the consistency of honey. Let it cool overnight to form crystals of salt, then separate them from their juice. Pour fresh water over the crystals and evaporate as before, then pour out the water or juice, mix it with the first, and cook them together until they thicken. Let the mixture cool for two days to form new crystals, then add them to the first batch. Repeat this process until the crystals of salt no longer form.

Dessicate and calcine all of the salt in an earthenware crucible in the furnace of calcination, taking care not to melt the crystals. After calcined to whiteness, pour the salt in the rectified *aqua vitae* already obtained and distill seven times, slowly, as previously instructed. This ardent spirit dissolves gold that has been prepared according to the art, but it must circulate at length before it becomes homogenous with its menstruum. This path is shorter than the former and gives equally good results, although the previous method is the way of the sages and requires great subtlety, patience, and skill.

Distillation *per descensum*

This method of distillation is poorly known but necessary to obtain the essential oils of juniper, herb bennet, nutmeg, and several other plants. The procedure requires a square furnace made of uncooked bricks, measuring three cubits on each side and one and a half cubits high on the exterior. It must be consolidated by fittings and at its upper median part there should be a hole one foot in diameter. The hearth should have a shelter made of walled tiles that is high enough to cover several cucurbits at a time, and the furnace should be clean before the operation begins.

Use one or two cucurbits, either earthenware or of tinned copper, although one will likely suffice. The substance to be distilled must not occupy more than one-third of the volume of the cucurbit. Cover the cucurbit with a tinplate lid pierced with small holes, then invert it, with the top at the bottom and the bottom at the top, so that its neck passes through the hole formed in the bottom of the stove, which should measure three fingers in width.

Adapt the receptacle to the lower part of the furnace to receive the distilling matter and fire the upper part of the furnace with coal on all sides, but at as far a remove as possible from the distillatory. Gradually increase the fire, which should be small in the beginning. Since the water will be first to exit, in a greater or lesser quantity depending on the plant matter in question, place a glass cucurbit in the lower part of the furnace, under the orifice of the upper bottom, to receive the distillate. Once the distilling oil appears, empty this vessel, and do so again, if necessary, as the fire is made stronger and moved closer to the distillatory. Continue until the oil no longer distills. Next, set the fire back as much as possible and let it go out, allowing the top of the cucurbit to cool down. Immediately remove the lower part containing the oil and preserve it separately, for this oil is subtle, essential, balsamic, and well suited to noble pursuits.

Quintessence of Greater Celandine

There are two species of celandine, greater celandine and lesser celandine. The virtues of both are unimaginable when they have been made to yield their quintessence, which requires both a subtle artistry and a significant amount of time. Gather a quantity of greater celandine when it is ripe, green, and beginning to whiten, and be sure to harvest the whole plant. Chop the plants into pieces and crush them in a mortar. Put them in a glass cucurbit, make sure it is well sealed and well luted, and set it in the steam bath or let it ferment for three weeks.

Adapt the alembic and set it to distill in the water bath with a very slow fire until the water comes out. Draw the residue and finely grind it in a marble mortar, then return it to the vessel together with its water, place the blind alembic on top, and lute them together. Putrefy the matter in the water bath for seven days, then in the ash bath with the beak alembic, then distill as instructed in the example above concerning the separation of earth and oil. A clear water having the color of oil will then emerge. This water will contain the elements Air and Water; the elements Earth and Fire will remain at the bottom of the vessel. To separate the phlegm from the oil, distill it in the water bath with a slow fire. The oil alone will remain, and the Air and the Water will be separated.

To obtain the elements Fire and Earth, grind the residue in a marble mortar, combine it with four times as much of its phlegm, and bathe it for seven days. Afterward, distill it in the sand bath at a high heat, until a red water ascends and exits completely. This red water contains the elements Fire and Water, and the element Earth, which is black in color, will remain at the bottom of the vessel. Next, distill the red water in another cucurbit in the water bath with a beak alembic, and when all the phlegm has gone out, a red oil will remain at the bottom of the vessel, which is the element Fire, and thus the practitioner will have materialized each of the four elements. Dessicate and calcine the earth for ten days, grind it and mix it with four times as much of its phlegm, then distill it through the alembic until small white stones like salt appear. Dissolve this salt in the distilled water and redistill. Then dissolve and distill once more until the earth becomes white like wax. Lastly, conclude the operation by rectifying the earth.

To use the elements, each of them must circulate in the water bath for thirty days with four parts earth. The quintessence, which will float over the matter, should be distilled very slowly so that it becomes perfect and pure: this is the soul of the greater celandine.

The phlegm or Water is good for hot or cold maladies, tempers the veins and the arteries, purifies the blood, cures diseases of the bronchi, and protects against all corruptions. The oil or Air rejuvenates and comforts and destroys black and yellow bile with an admirably temperate action. The spirit, Fire, or quintessence, when taken at a dose of 1 grain dissolved in a good Spanish wine and applied to the neck and chest of subjects who are seriously ill, will restore their health and vigor in a short amount of time, for it penetrates to the heart, which it purifies and vivifies instantaneously. Even if the practitioner wishes to resuscitate the terminally ill, life will be restored to them, according to Pseudo-Llull, if they absorb a like quantity of dissolved quintessence.[15] This medicine, however, should never be administered in cases of violent or hot fevers.

Extracting the Quintessence from Fruits

Cut the fruits into pieces and pound them in an earthenware mortar with a tenth part of cleaned salt. Put them in a cucurbit with a well-luted blind alembic and digest them in the steam bath of water or lime. After fifteen or thirty days, when the juice starts to float over the feces, begin the distillations using the Philipp Ulstad method of extracting the quintessence from plants, but with the following exception: the salt must be extracted and the circulation made only with the desiccated and pulverized residue.

This quintessence is refreshing and comforting and serves as an excellent cure for hot or bilious maladies.*

Quintessence of Honey

Put some thick pink honey in an iron cauldron with an equal portion of fountain water and cook with a slow heat, skimming off the surface when it becomes covered a total of nine times. The mixture should be made to the original consistency of the honey. Next, put this honey in a circulatory vessel in a water bath of the first degree for forty days. At the end of the philosophical month, put it in a tall and long glass cucurbit and distill it through the alembic. If the honey does not show, the practitioner must surround the cucurbit with wet cloths until the clear water comes out. Preserve this water separately, because it is an excellent formula for regrowing hair. After this, a second, golden-colored water will ascend. Preserve this water separately, too, because it may be used

---

*The quintessence of golden reinette apple is especially sovereign.

for healing wounds or coloring hair. Once this water has exited, distill what remains in the ash bath, and as soon as it begins to redden and brown, preserve this third water separately. However, to obtain the maximum virtue of the honey, circulate these three waters together for seven days and distill them three times over their feces. At the fourth distillation, set aside the first liquor, which should amount to one-half of the whole mixture, then redistill the remaining half four times according to the art.

Quintessence of Aromatic Plants

Put 32 pounds of excellent white wine in the bain-marie and distill until it reduces to 6 or 8 pounds. Repeat the same procedure with another white wine and continue until you obtain 32 pounds of spirit of distilled wine. Put this spirit in the distillatory and set it under a slow fire until the spirit reduces by half. Pour the spirit into a cucurbit and distill until all the phlegm is removed, then redistill four more times in the water bath. After the fourth distillation, add 1 dram each of aloeswood, cardamom, and fresh cubeb pepper and 4 drams each of cinnamon, nutmeg, white ginger, long pepper, grains of paradise, and sandalwood, all of which should be finely pulverized. Put the mixture in a well-sealed glass vessel in the water bath for eight days and distill it through the alembic with a slow fire. Transfer the mixture to a long-necked matrass with 2 drams each of finely pulverized cloves and ambergris, seal the matrass, and put it in the water bath for a fortnight over a gentle and continuous heat. Next, separate the liquor from the feces and distill it three times with a slow fire. At the end of the third distillation, use a stronger fire and then allow the liquor to cool. This is a quintessence of the second order.

To obtain a quintessence of the first order, draw out the feces and dry them in an earthenware vessel over a high heat. When they become brittle, mix them well with the liquor, put them in the circulatory for seven days, and distill the liquor four times over its feces, which should be dried before each distillation. Then, finally, distill or rectify the liquor three times by itself with a slow fire. There is not a single wet or cold disease this quintessence cannot cure.

Paracelsus's *Elixir proprietatis*

Pulverize together 4 ounces each of myrrh, aloe, and saffron. Put them in a glass vessel with a double portion of spirit of wine. Add to this mixture some oil of sulfur, previously made and rectified using the tin *campana* during a bout of rainy weather. The oil should float above the liquor at an eminence of three fingers. Digest everything for two days, circulating often, then decant the tincture and preserve it. Afterward, pour spirit of wine over the residue and digest the mixture for two months, circulating it every day in order to draw out the tincture. Reunite the first and second tinctures, then distill them together.

The virtues of this elixir are preventative, purifying, stomachic, pulmonary, and cordial. It not only prevents the onset of all diseases, but also prolongs life. Its dose is 6 to 12 drops in some white wine.*

Tincture of Coral

Take some hard, compressed, and bright red coral and reduce it to a fine powder. Put the powder in a matrass and pour over 2 ounces of the 1st menstruum (see below). Shake it immediately and then pour 2 more ounces of the 1st menstruum over the matter. Repeat, adding 2 ounces at a time up to an eminence of four inches. Adapt another matrass to make a circulatory vessel, lute it, and set it to digest in the steam bath made of chopped straw and quicklime for three weeks. Afterward, open the vessel, decant the tinted menstruum, and preserve it in a closed vessel. Pour more of the 1st menstruum over the remaining coral and continue digesting and extracting until the menstruum loses its color. Then join all the dyed waters together and filter them. Put them in a cucurbit in the sand bath and remove the phlegm or liquor with a moderate heat. At the bottom of the vessel there will remain a red powder that contains the true tincture and virtue of the coral.

Next, put this powder in a circulatory vessel or pelican and pour over six fingers of the 2nd menstruum (see below). Carefully lute the opening at the top of the vessel after sealing it with a glass stopper.

---

*This is Le Fèvre's version of Paracelsus's *elixir proprietatis* (see *Cours de la chymie*, 1:266–68), which, as we shall demonstrate in a separate study, is insufficiently spagyric.

Place this vessel in the bath and let it digest for forty days. The menstruum will gently draw to itself the admirable sulfur of the coral along with its tincture. Stop the fire, draw and filter the tincture, then put it in a cucurbit and distill off two-thirds. Preserve the rest with great care, as it is one of the most effective remedies of spagyric medicine.*

1st Menstruum: Mix 4 pounds of purified and pulverized tartar with 1 pound of vitriol of Mars.† Put this mixture in a large matrass and pour over 3 pounds of vitriolic water tinged with its volatile sulfurous spirit. Adapt it to another matrass to make a circulatory vessel, lute it, then set it to digest in the steam bath for seven days. Pour the product of the digestion into a cucurbit with one-half of its body luted with clay, cover it with a well-luted capital, and place it in the reverberatory furnace. Adapt a receptacle, the joints of which should be very smooth, and increase the fire gradually, by degrees, until the drops begin to follow each other successively. Maintain the fire at this degree until the drops no longer emerge. At this point, increase the fire gradually until all the vapors are gone and the capital clears up on its own, then quit the fire and let everything cool. Separate the distilled liquor from the tartar oil by filtering the mixture and rectify the spirit in the ash bath until dry. This menstruum is used to open up the coral without calcining it.

2nd Menstruum (aqua temperata): Mix together equal parts of alcohol of pure wine and spirit of dephlegmed salt, little by little, then distill them through the beak alembic in the ash bath four or five times until perfect union is achieved. This menstruum is used to extract the inner sulfur from the coral, which will still hide in the shadow of the body after using the 1st menstruum.[16]

---

*Although coral ultimately belongs to the mineral kingdom, we give the operation for extracting its tincture here because preparations of coral are now regularly included among homeopathic herbal remedies.

†[Vitriol of Mars (*vitriolum Martis*), a preparation of oil of vitriol and iron filings, is otherwise known as ferric sulphate, a white crystalline substance that forms a red solution when it is dissolved in water. —*Trans.*]

The Spagyric Art of Extracting Quintessences:
A Theoretical and Practical Synthesis

The operations described in this chapter are intended to shepherd students of Hermetic herbalism in the many different situations they are likely to encounter in the course of their studies. Each disease has its own particular treatment that requires the use of one or more plants, and the preparation of these plants will vary according to their genus, species, and elemental nature, as well as their planetary and zodiacal signature, and it is in this respect that the preceding examples will be most useful.

We could have included additional preparations from famous authors such as Oswald Croll, Jean François Fernel, David de Planis Campi, Sir Robert Boyle, Sir Kenelm Digby, or Father Gabriel de Castaigne, among others, but this would have added nothing to the Hermetic value of this chapter because the works of these authors, although well reputed, cannot hold a candle to the works of the spagyric masters that have guided our research. Nevertheless, out of fear that some students will consult such authors in the course of their studies and, as a result, fail to draw from them sufficiently well-grounded and spagyric notions and procedures, we thought it wise to summarize the principles and practice of spagyrics in a concise and precise synthesis that may serve as a guide in the majority of cases.

All mixed bodies are formed of the union of an active-vital substance and a passive-neutral matter, which are the soul and body, the spirit and matter, the pure and impure. Both life and virtue are contained in the essential substance that animates corporeal matter, which in turn restrains and fixes the substance. To extract the pure active principle from any plant, the practitioner must separate the essential substance from its material body spagyrically, for this impure and crude body impedes its soul and restrains it, to the point of neutralizing its action.

The soul attains its maximum virtue only when it has been separated from its body. To perform this separation in a natural manner, the artist must break down the mixed body into its primitive elements by retrogression: this is what the ancients called *reincruding* matter. In spagyrics, involution or the return of matter to its first principles always precedes evolution, for all generation is born of putrefaction.

Putrefaction is generated by a *warm moisture* of the nature of spring, which corrupts seeds and reincrudes them before they can germinate and vegetate. The retrogression of the mixed body to its elemental matter is nothing less than the destruction of its form by a return to the primitive chaos. This chaos is the primordial water which contains the elements of life and form in an embryonic state. First and foremost, it is therefore necessary to corrupt mixed bodies by the *warm moisture* that causes *putrefaction* and in this manner to dissolve them in their elemental water. What follows is a general succession of the spagyric operations performed on plants.

Take a certain quantity of a fresh plant and chop it into small pieces. Put them in a sealed glass vessel or matrass with some carefully filtered rainwater, such that its contents do not exceed half the capacity of the matrass. Subject this well-luted and well-sealed vessel to the uniform action of a slow and humid heat for forty days. At the end of the philosophical month the plant matter, having lost its form, will be dissolved in a chaotic water. Separate this water from the residue by a weak expression and then clarify it by filtration. Next, put the water in a vessel with a fresh supply of the same plant, prepared in the same manner as before, and ferment or putrefy the whole mixture with the same humid heat for thirty days. Separate and filter the newly obtained water and digest it for eight days in the water bath. Distill this water according to the rules of the art with a gentle and regular fire, so that the matter distills slowly and without agitation. Increase the degree of the fire gradually when its action abates—this must be done with prudence and subtlety, as we have instructed.

Draw out all the phlegm or insipid water and set it apart so that the spirit may distill without mixing. Once the spirit has been distilled and set aside, heat the fire in order to raise the oil or essence and collect it separately. When this process has been completed, extract the residue from the vessel and burn it gradually between two crucibles, one inverted upon the other, until it is reduced to a white ash. Dissolve this ash in the phlegm drawn from the previous distillation, then filter and evaporate this solution in a large and flat vessel, at the bottom of which the crystalline salt will appear. Wash and dissolve this salt in clarified rainwater and evaporate it to obtain a pure and diaphanous salt. Having reached this stage of the work, the practitioner will possess the three constituent principles of the separated plant: the spirit or Mercury, the essence or Sulfur, and the saline principle or Salt.

The spirit must be rectified by repeated distillations until it is pure and subtle; the essence and the salt must ennoble each other. Dissolve the salt in the essential oil and circulate the solution in the pelican with a slow heat for fifteen days or until the oil is impregnated with the volatile part of the salt. This essence must be rectified by repeated distillations until it becomes light and pure. All that remains, then, is to add it to its spirit. To do this, combine the spirit and the essence in the circulatory of Hermes and subject it to a gentle heat for fifteen days so that the spirit and the oil are inseparably united, each one to the other, in a single liquor, then rectify it three times. This liquor is a true quintessence, since it is formed of the union of the three constituent principles of the mixed body, namely Mercury (the spirit) and Sulfur (the oil) united by (the volatile) Salt. Every quintessence, in fact, should be formed of a unity of these three principles and not just the spirit alone, as many erroneously believe.

This work is long and arduous and requires a great deal of patience and diligence. Unlike moderns, the ancients lived modestly and had pure and simple customs. They could devote themselves to achieving holy and noble works because their way of life was not cluttered with the useless baggage of conventions, contingencies, and frivolous habits.

To close this chapter, we shall reaffirm the assertions of the judicious Guy de la Brosse, namely that not all parts of mixed bodies possess an equal virtue, and that to prepare anodyne remedies, practitioners must separate from the body of the plant that organ wherein its chief virtue resides.[17] However, since the quintessence is imprinted with the astral nature of the plant from which it is extracted, and since this astral nature is equally distributed throughout the entire body of the plant, it is advisable for practitioners to operate on the body *in the state in which it is found at the time of harvest,* according to its genus and species.

PART THREE

HELMONTIAN MEDICINE AND THE PREPARATION OF ALKAHESTS AND MENSTRUAL VEHICLES

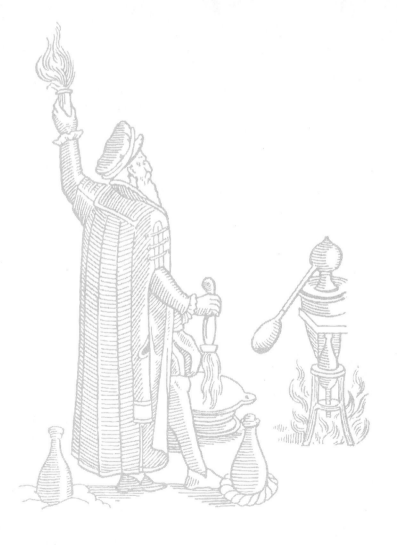

16

The Spagyric Medicines
of Paracelsus and Helmont

Now that we have offered brief descriptions of the preparations of ordinary chemistry and a thorough study of the operations of spagyric chemistry, the time is ripe to elucidate the philosophical works of another disciple of Paracelsus, namely Jan Baptist van Helmont (1580–1644), whose theories were highly influential. Helmont was both a learned doctor and a sincere man, but he went astray in two essential ways: he placed far too much confidence in his own doctrine, and he never acquired the key to the Hermetic Sanctuary.

Initially, Helmont was a declared adversary of alchemy, but he became convinced of its validity when an unknown adept performed a transmutation before his very eyes.[1] The preparation of remedies by means of the *alkahest* or "universal solvent" came to form the basis of Helmont's works. He averred that with the aid of the alkahest he could reduce any mixed body to its constituent principles, each one separate from the other, while preserving the vegetative virtue in their seed.

Helmont claimed he had discovered the great alkahest of Paracelsus, but the latter never spoke of this alkahest save in a few very brief and uninformative remarks. Elsewhere Paracelsus speaks of several arcana having the same properties as the alkahest, but without ever designating them by this name. Helmont was as silent as Paracelsus on the subject of the alkahest's composition, and one wonders whether he was truly in possession of this particular arcanum or if he only knew of something similar.

Even though Helmont never revealed the formula for his alkahest, he still recommended, in the absence of this arcanum, the use of volatilized alkalis, and he advised practitioners to esteem among all of the salts that of tartar as the best and most penetrating. According to Helmont, this salt when volatilized is equal in virtue to the greatest arcana because of its resolutive and detersive properties and because it is capable of penetrating the human organism and resolving the excremental humors and any unnatural coagulation it encounters in the vessels, even after a fourth digestion. Salt of tartar purifies the blood and unblocks even the most obstinate obstructions, thus dissipating the material causes of diseases. Its spirit is so penetrating and active that its ability to cleanse the body of all impurities is inestimable. The spirit of these volatile salts has an admirable resolutive quality that can dissolve all simples and, upon coagulation, take on their specific virtue, curing the most stubborn maladies and fevers in the human body.

What follows is a summary exposition of Helmont's doctrine concerning volatile alkalis, a doctrine which, according to the testimony of several of his disciples, and George Starkey among them, is both tried and true.

Summary of Helmont's Preparations

Among the processes that Helmont suggests for the volatilization of alkalis, one of the best is his preparation with vegetable oils *drawn by expression*. When boiled in alkali detergents, these oils will form a soap that contains little volatile salt in itself, but its *caput mortuum* will contain a large quantity of fixed salt. Essential or distilled oils cannot, due to their volatility, be boiled with detergents to make soap. But there exists, according to Helmont, a more secret way by which these oils and the salt of tartar can be made, not into a soap, but into a volatile diaphanous salt that dissolves in water or wine. In this operation, one part alkali will turn two or three parts oil into pure salt, without any oleaginousness, with the exception of a small portion of oil that turns into a resinous gum distinct from the salt.

This salt dissolves like any other salt. If the solution is evaporated to the cuticle, it will crystallize in the color of the plant from which the oil was extracted. This salt is so mortified and mild that one can hold it on one's tongue without the slightest inconvenience. The distilled oils, although hot and pungent to the taste, retain in this operation only so much taste and smell as is inseparable from the *viva media* or the average life of the mixed body, so that the medicine is temperate, diuretic, and insensibly diaphoretic. Salts made in this manner are perfectly volatile, without leaving any fixed salt in the dead earth or *caput mortuum.*

This operation can be easily performed in two months' time and render sufficient quantities, provided it is done according to Helmont's instruction, that is, *sine aqua, occulta et artificiosa circulatione,* or to speak more plainly, as long as the digestion is made *in the deepest center of matter.*

The heat required must never exceed that of the Sun in spring, in which heat alone, by spagyric art, the salt receives a fermentative determination from the oils, while the oils receive the same from the salt. Thus, from the two is born a volatile temperate salt possessing the virtue of each parent substance, for it receives a diuretic and detersive virtue from the alkali and a balsamic virtue from the oil, which is capable of penetrating our constitutive principles. This salt, once elixirated, is so volatile that it can be dissolved or cooked in water without losing its virtue.

This elixir is an "absolute corrector" of the venoms in all poisonous plants, which it mortifies immediately, so that stinking hellebore, monkshood, henbane, and squirting cucumber, among other poisonous plants, simply by mixing with this volatile tartar, suddenly become innocuous, and this is done at a temperature close to that of the human body. In a short but very artificial digestion, the practitioner can use this elixir to obtain volatile salts from herbs that do not render any essential oil when they are distilled with water such as stinking hellebore, jalap, bryony, and elecampane, among others, which become salutary remedies when corrected in this manner, for besides having their own particular properties, they also take on those of the elixir with which they are united. The elixir on its own is a balsamic *ens* of admirable efficacy in dire cases. According to Starkey, author of *Nature's Explication and Helmont's Vindication:*

Whoever, then, wants to become a true child of the Art should learn to use salts according to their true philosophical preparation and not by their ordinary preparations, in which they are simply extracted from the ashes of plants by depuration and then filtered and coagulated, for in this state they cannot go beyond a second digestion. But when they are volatilized, they become balsamic tinctures and familiar to our nature, and so are easily admitted to have entrance even to our constitutive principles, according to the nature of the concrete whose *crasis* resides in its volatility.[2]

Treatment of Alkalis

George Starkey, who provides much useful information on the manufacture of volatile alkalis, was one of Helmont's greatest champions. The following summary exposition expresses his own opinions on the treatment of alkalis.

There are two ways to volatilize alkalis, by alcoholization and by elixiration. Alcoholization is the circulation of a fixed alkali with a volatile spirit until the two become one and a neutral production arises that is distinct from each parent substance. Now, there are three distinct kinds of spirits, namely acid spirits, alkaline spirits, and vinous spirits, which make three distinct kinds of alcoholized alkalis, namely the *arcanum ponticitatis, arcanum microcismi,* and *arcanum samech.* Elixiration is performed by essential or distilled oils or tinctures until the two parent substances produce a volatile salt that possesses the nature of the particular oil or tincture.

Of these various operations, the easiest to perform is the *arcanum ponticitatis,* which consists in producing an ebullition by pouring an acid on an alkali until it is saturated, a process which destroys the igneous corrosion of the alkali and makes it volatile. This result is obtained by repeated cohobation of the acid on the alkali, which after ebullition is mixed with burnt clay and distilled in the manner of the spirit of salt or niter, until nothing else distills. It is then necessary to cohobate a new acid spirit on the *caput mortuum* until it is satiated, then to distill it a second time with a very strong fire, repeating this work until all of the alkali ascends with the acid spirit. This can be done with the spirit of vitriol, salt, or niter or with distilled vinegar, the result of which is an *acetum forte* or *acetum radicis,* as Paracelsus calls it.

But there is another way that does not require distillation. It is sufficient to imbibe the alkali with a spirit until it produces a neutral salt, which the practitioner may then dephlegmate and join with the rectified tincture of any plant, digesting them until they crystallize in the form of a colored salt, which contains "the *crasis* of the concrete."³

There are other more effective preparations, of which we shall give our readers some glimpses. It should be noted, however, that the acidity of the spirit of niter and the spirit of vitriol is very different from the acidity of the stomach, which is a fermentative principle. It is necessary, then, to find a means by which the nature of the former can be transformed into the nature the latter, because the stomach acid can extinguish the igneous nature of an alkali if the remedy does not possess excess quantities of the alkali and the alkali is not of a mineral nature. Therefore, practitioners must exercise caution with salts that have mineral origins, as their preparation requires exceptional skill on the part of the artist.

To summarize, the practitioner must succeed in producing a very pure and neutral salt without any bitterness, which, over the course of prolonged digestion and circulation with the essence of the mixed body, becomes anodyne, mild, and subtle, and which, by its volatility, exalts the virtue of the mixed body and penetrates the human organism along with it, even after the final digestions. The best way to achieve volatilization is by essential oils or by vinous spirits that are volatile sulfurs of a more ennobled nature than that of the mineral acids. They must conjoin "without any water, by a secret and artificial circulation" (*sine aqua, occulta et artificiosa circulatione*). If this is accomplished, they will transform into volatile salt in the space of three months. Alkalis and essential oils thus prepared will embrace each other in bonds of love having the smell of ammonia and the consistency of a soapy cream.

The practitioner must continue the decoction until the mixture dissolves in spirit of wine without raising any fat to the surface, that is, until the spirit unites intimately and inseparably with the mixture. When this solution is rectified with a moderate heat, a burning volatile spirit having the taste and smell of the oil will ascend first. The insipid phlegm will ascend next, and the dyed balsamic elixir will remain at the bottom of the vessel. After dephlegmating the spirit, unite it with this elixir and digest them together until perfect union is achieved. To obtain a perfect elixir, however, it must be dried and crystallized without any additives or any separative culinary heat and nourished with its oil until it imbibes three times its own quantity. Air will engender the cold and the dry, and Fire—*not vulgar fire*—will generate the hot and the wet. Understand this well and the secret of the alkahest and the mysteries of the Sun and Mercury shall be revealed to you.

17
The Art of Volatilizing Alkalis

To aid researchers in the art of volatilizing alkalis, we offer here a compilation of some of the best procedures.

Volatilizing Salt of Tartar: Method 1

Dissolve some very white salt of tartar in distilled vinegar, then filter and evaporate until a film develops on the surface. Mix in twice as much fine white sand and reverberate them together for twelve hours in an unglazed earthenware vessel. Redissolve the reverberated salt in vinegar, then filter, evaporate, reverberate, and dissolve until the salt of tartar becomes white as snow.

Redissolve this salt in distilled vinegar and evaporate the mixture in the water bath, then dissolve it once more until the vinegar becomes sharp and pungent. Dry the salt slowly, then add to it an equal measure of spirit of wine and digest them together. Distill them over a slow heat, then add more spirit and digest once more. Repeat this procedure until the spirit of wine comes out as strong as it was prior to its use, then evaporate gently. Sublimate the salt by fire and preserve it in a sealed vessel.

Volatilizing Salt of Tartar: Method 2

Mix pure salt of tartar with its spirit until it is completely saturated, then put the mixture in a glass matrass, lute its head and receiver well, and distill until desiccated. Extract what little fixed salt remains in the matrass after the distillation and calcine it in a crucible with the fire of fusion.

Put this salt back into the matrass and cohobate it with the liquor drawn from the distillation. Distill again in the same manner as before and repeat this operation until the fixed salt absorbs all of the spirit of tartar, which should occur during the seventh distillation. Pour rectified wine over the prepared salt and distill them until the fixed salt absorbs all of the spirit of wine.

Volatilizing Salt of Tartar: Method 3

Grind separately 1 pound each of salt of tartar and saltpeter and mix them together. Put the mixture in a clean iron pot, set it over the coal fire, and stir the material with an iron rod until the red color disappears and the salt becomes very white. To obtain the alkali of pure tartar, calcine it in the furnace until it forms into a white mass, then put the tartar calcined by the niter in a crucible in the wind furnace until it melts. Next, pour it into a preheated bronze mortar and dissolve it into a bluish alkaline mass, which will dissolve in the air. Take this calcined salt and dissolve it by stirring it in boiling water, then let stand until it clarifies and the remaining impurities settle at the bottom. Gently pour out the clear liquid and evaporate until dry.

To obtain a batch that is perfectly pure, take the solution of one of the salts before its evaporation and mix it with an equal portion of clear lime in water. Allow them to ferment for a fortnight in a covered stoneware vessel, then pour out the clear liquid, evaporate until dry in a clean vessel, and you will obtain a pure white volatile salt. After obtaining the volatile salt, digest it slowly with the expressed oil of the desired plant. According to Helmont, this digestion must be long and protracted and end with a thorough circulation in order to revolatilize the salt obtained.

Digest this salt with spirit of wine at a very gentle heat and it will take on the tincture of the plant. After several digestions the salt will be stripped of its tincture. At this stage, all that remains is to distill the spirit at a slow heat and it will leave the tincture at the bottom of the vessel. This tincture is the pure *crasis* of the plant and serves as an excellent remedy.

Preparation of the Samech Elixir

Starkey speaks of a certain Samech elixir obtained by the union of alkalis volatilized by essential oils with alkalis volatilized by spirit of wine. The basis of the operation is the distillation and cohobation of oil of terebinth with a mineral sulfur until perfect union is achieved. Once elixirated, mix in salt of tartar and extract the tincture with spirit of wine.

Dissolve the Samech in spirit of wine enriched with cinnamon, then distill and separate the spirit. Dephlegmate the spirit and the Samech, then reunite them, mixing them intimately together. Next, take saffron, myrrh, or aloe, or all three together, reduce them to a powder and mix in an equal portion of tartar, then digest by means of an artificial digestion that is so active they yield their full, corrected, and exalted tincture. Add to the Samech elixir both the tincture extracted and the spirit of wine enriched with cinnamon and draw the spirit, which will possess a marvelous sweet-smelling aroma. The balm and the spirit, when reunited by a secret digestion, will make a *Samech elixiris proprietatis* that is extremely fragrant and will equal, if not exceed, the preparation using the alkahest. To increase the virtue of this elixir, bring it first to a spontaneous granulation by degrees until achieving complete desiccation. Nourish it afterward with an aromatic spirit six to eight times, each time drying it in the air and moistening it with a moderate fire of sand. After sublimation, you will have the Samech, the elixirated oils, and the glorified tinctures all sublimated together. Its virtues are admirable and manifold. Its dose is from 10 to 20 grains.

The same procedure may be used to prepare all sorts of vegetable tinctures. For example, to make an eminent splenic or cephalic, use hellebore prepared with wild ginger root and jalap, or jalap and opium. For a hepatic, use elecampane root prepared with rhubarb and horseradish. To make a stomachic, use saffron, rosemary flowers, and bistort root. For a powerful diaphoretic, use bistort root, saffron, and opium. To make an eminent diuretic, use rhubarb, saffron, and satyrion, which both Paracelsus and Helmont used to make their *Aroph*, that is, *aro(ma) ph(ilosophorum)* or "philosophers' aroma." For a good laxative, use colocynth, aloe, and balsam of Peru. To combat coughs or dysentery, use opium, caranna, and brindleberry. The practitioner, of course, may use different ingredients and compose other herbal remedies as reason directs, according to the nature of the plants and the nature of the illness in need of treatment.[1]

Helmont's Alkahest
and Alkahests in General

An investigation into question of Helmont's alkahest will lead us into discussions of the solvents of the masters. First, however, we may solve radically at least one aspect of this question: there can be only one *universal* solvent, which is the Mercury of the Philosophers, and since Helmont did not know its composition, his alkahest can only be a *particular* solvent. The confidence he had in this particular solvent and the enthusiasm he showed for all that he discovered made him exaggerate the virtues of his alkahest, whose formulation he never revealed.

Here is what Starkey has to say about it in *Pyrotechny Asserted and Illustrated:*

> When the alkahest resolves plants into their first liquid matter, it distinguishes them in all their heterogeneities, in which resolution there always seats itself in a distinct place a small amount of liquor, eminently distinguishable from the rest in color, in which the *crasis* of the mixed resides. Therefore, the most desirable and truly philosophical way to perform this is by the addition of an agent which is penetrative and fermentative, so that it dissolves the mixed without any altering or sensible heat by a secret circulation. For when we dissolve a simple that renders its oil, the oil separates from the mercurial liquor, and the oil and the liquor separate from the solvent to be digested by the same heat into a salt, which is the *primum ens* of the plant. The alkahest can be separated from the body it has dissolved, and the remedy prepared will possess only the virtue—but more precise and exalted—of the mixed body from which it was made, while the volatile alkali will remain united to the balsamic tincture of the oil it volatilized and to the essences of whichever herbs were added to it, enhancing their medicinal virtues.[2]

And so, unbeknownst to Helmont, the virtues he ascribed to his alka-hest are the same as those which the sages ascribed to their Philosophical Mercury. What, then, are we to conclude from all this?

Despite the cloud of obscurity that hangs over the composition of the alkahest, whether Paracelsus's or Helmont's, it is not impossible for the practitioner *on the true path* to penetrate its particular nature, as we shall try to demonstrate. Most authors believe the alkahest to be a volatile and supremely exalted alkali. Sieur Jean Le Pelletier of Rouen, however, published a treatise in which he suggests that the alkahest is a product of human urine.[3] What error and candor! Are we really to believe that the *universal arcanum* may be drawn from mammalian matter?

The first use of the term "alkahest" appears in the second book of Paracelsus's *De viribus membrorum:*

> There is also the liquor alkahest, of great efficacy in preserving the liver, and also in curing all other diseases arising from disorders of that part of the body. It must be resolved after its coagulation and coagulated again into a transmutated form, as the process of coagu-lation and resolution teaches, for once it has surmounted its like, it becomes superior to all other hepatic medicines, and even if the liver were broken and dissolved, this medicine would stand in the place of the whole liver.[4]

And that's all Paracelsus had to say about the alkahest. Nevertheless, from this very same passage Helmont concluded that the alkahest was a certain *sals circulatum* that Paracelsus elsewhere calls the *circulatum majus* or "greater circulation." Now, it is indeed possible to draw a powerful solvent from common salt or niter by repeated resolution and circulation, but this cannot be the alkahest of which Helmont speaks because all arcana having universal properties can only be found in the metallic kingdom, and this is precisely what led Gerhard Dorn and Martin Ruland to conclude that the alkahest of Paracelsus was a "pre-pared mercury."[5] From this it follows that the Helmontian alkahest cannot be identical with the Paracelsian alkahest.

Helmont spoke obscurely of an antimony-based preparation that consisted in extracting the mercurial principle from this mineral and dissolving it in the essence of exalted terebinth by repeated circulation and sublimation. After achieving a perfect union, it was necessary to dissolve this product in an alkahest of niter and to circulate them together until they no longer made a single body. We believe spirit of wine intervened in the purification of this mineral menstruum, which, in point of fact, possesses some of the virtues that Helmont attributes to the alkahest. There are, however, much more plausible candidates for the alkahest among the solvents and menstrua employed by Pseudo-Llull and Paracelsus.

First of all, to obtain an alkahest worthy of the name, the practitioner must possess the saline alkahests of tartar, niter, and common salt, by which the mercurial substance of certain metals may be intimately dissolved. Still, none of these menstrua equals the virtue of the Mercury of the Philosophers, but since this subject is solely the prerogative of the children of Hermes, we shall not divulge it here. In addition to the three aforementioned saline menstrua, the practitioner must know how to extract a divine spirit from thunderstorm water, by which *all mineral menstrua* may be ennobled spagyrically. The spirit of wine, subtilized and exalted using the methods previously described, is a powerful agent of purification and acuity in the preparation of menstrua. These are the five spirits required in the work of alkahests. This composition has always been secret, and we unveil it here for the first time. But this work, it must be stressed, can be accomplished only by *spagyric artistry,* which is to say, it cannot be achieved by vulgar chemistry. Therefore, we advise readers to meditate at length upon all we have said above—and will say below—concerning this philosophical art.

In addition to these five spirits or first menstrua, the work of alkahests requires the cooperation of certain mercurial metals, because there can be no alkahest *outside the mineral kingdom.* These metallic elements are lead, antimony, mercury, tin, and, lastly, the *metallus primus,* the noblest metal of all. The latter is the same metal used by Paracelsus, but we leave it to researchers to discover its true identity. The first three saline spirits are active at first and must be subtilized by the *quintessence of wine,* then ennobled, attenuated, and evolved by the *spirit drawn from rainwater.*

Quintessence of Salts

To extract the quintessence from salts like common salt, salt niter, antimony, or vitriol, Paracelsus provides the following instruction in *De viribus membrorum:* "Cohobate them frequently with their own proper liquid or with water, putrefy with phlegm, and abstract the body from thence after the manner of phlegm, even to the fixed spirit. This dissolve in water or its proper liquid, and separate in heat, with spirit of wine, the pure from the impure."[6]

A philosophical menstruum should never be corrosive like vulgar *aquae fortes* since its function is to fortify, preserve, purify, exalt, and separate the soul from the body, not to destroy as the strong waters do. At this point we would advise readers to ponder what we have said concerning the cold fires. Saline spirits should serve as *active principles* only during the beginning of the operation, after which their destructive and corrosive nature must be diminished and modified to acquire a nobler, subtler, and more permanent latitude. What we have said concerning the volatilization of tartar should suffice to extract a subtle solvent, but as for common salt and niter, we shall speak plainly enough that the wise disciple may be in a position to extract the quintessence. What follows is an operative procedure for making an alkahest from common salt, which Paracelsus calls the *circulatum minus* or "lesser circulation":

Calcine four times some common salt decrepitated with an equal portion of powdered quicklime, the first time for four hours, then decrease each subsequent calcination by one hour. Dissolve it in plenty of water, filter, and coagulate between each distillation. Pour seven parts spirit of salt on one part prepared salt and digest until dissolved, then put everything in the steam bath for thirty days and let it putrefy. Distill, separating the phlegm that ascends first, and pour the strongest spirit back over the gold-colored matter, which will turn red. Dissolve and putrefy as before until the matter resembles a red oil. This is the quintessence of common salt.

To subtilize it still further and deprive it of all bitterness, circulate it with spirit of wine and distill by cohobating the spirit over the residue several times. To exalt it, draw the phlegm and then the element Air (or oil), by which it is necessary to extract the element Fire remaining at the bottom. Initiates, however, know of a marvelous separator by which the phlegm may be flushed that cuts the duration of this procedure in half. The influence of spirit of rainwater must intervene next.

Alkahest of Niter

Dissolve salt niter in thunderstorm water clarified by the sand bath and evaporate several times until the niter loses its bitterness and odor. Put it in a melting crucible in the fire of fusion, adding pieces of coal little by little, as and when they ignite, which must be done repeatedly for two or three hours until the niter is fixed and greenish in color. Grind it into a fine powder and dissolve it in water by deliquium in the cellar, then filter, coagulate, and dry it. Pulverize it again and dissolve one part in four parts of dephlegmated niter spirit. Let it come to a boil and digest it in the ash bath, then add more spirit and redigest. Do this three times in all. Next, calcine the matter in the wheel of fire (*ignis rota*) for two or three hours until it becomes ruby red in color. To draw out the spirit, pulverize the matter and putrefy it in several vessels in the steam bath until it smells of sulfur and the spirits begin to ascend. Distill it in the water bath to remove the phlegm, then in the ash bath to obtain the spirit. When this part of the operation is complete, the practitioner will have the elements Fire, Water, and Air.

To obtain the element Earth, calcine the feces with the ardent mirror or a strong fire (*ignis fortis*), dissolve them in their water, then filter and crystallize. Dissolve the crystals in their spirit at a ratio of one part crystals to four parts spirit and digest, then cohobate until everything passes into an exuberant mercurial spirit, which must be cooked in the athanor until it passes through various colors. Treat this liquor with spirit of wine in the manner previously described. As in the above example concerning the spirit of common salt, the practitioner must ennoble this menstruum with spirit of rainwater, *by which it is made into an alkahest.**

---

*The quintessences of salt and niter have nothing in common with the ordinary spirits of these salts.

Separation of the Elements from Metals

Take saltpeter, vitriol, and alum in equal parts and distill them into an *aqua fortis*. Cohobate the distilled water several times on its feces, then distill it again in a glass vessel. Clarify a small amount of silver in this *aqua fortis* to attenuate it, then separate it after precipitating it with sal ammoniac.* Next, take your metal of choice in the form of granulated shot and dissolve it in this water. Afterward, separate it in the water bath and cohobate it several times on its residue until an oil forms at the bottom of the vessel. The color of the oil will depend on the practitioner's choice of metal: gold (☉) will turn the oil a light and brilliant red; silver (☾), a light azure; iron (♂), a dark red or garnet; copper (♀), a bright green; mercury (☿), a bright white; lead (♄), a livid gray; and tin (♃), a luteous or xanthous color.[7]

The metals in this operation divide into two distinct parts, the quintessence and the body, both of which take the form of a thick and viscous liquid. After their separation they can no longer be conjoined. The greasy oil of the impure body will be whitish in color, while the quintessential oil, as Paracelsus explains, will be colored by the tincture of the metal. In addition to the above procedure, Paracelsus describes another for extracting the quintessence from metals:

Dissolve the metal in water and distill this solution in the bath. Cohobate and putrefy it until it reduces to a thick oil. Distill the oil from small vials and cucurbits by means of an alembic, and one part of the metal will remain at the bottom. Reduce this to an oil as before and distill until everything reduces to oil. Let it putrefy for a month, then distill it again for an extended period of time with a slow fire. The vapors will ascend and fall into the receiver. Remove these vapors and two obscure colors will ascend, one white and the other depending on the nature and condition of the metal. They will ascend together but become separated in the receiver: the quintessence will remain at the bottom, and the impure white color will float above it. Separate them with a funnel and preserve the quintessence, over which pour rectified

---

*Pseudo-Llull suggests that the sal ammoniac used in this operation is a "quintessence of mercury."

spirit of wine and digest them together until the acidity separates from the metallic essence. Repeat this procedure until you no longer perceive any sharpness. Finally, pour over some water, distill, and wash until it is brought to its proper sweetness, then preserve it.[8]

This operation is obviously incomplete and ill-suited for the extraction of pure quintessences from metals. Nonetheless, it may serve to guide the student in the preparation of alkahests, which requires the mercurial principle of one of the five aforementioned metals. To summarize, the work of alkahests consists in obtaining the subtle and essential menstrual spirit of one of the three designated salts, dissolving one of the five mercurial metals (after preliminary preparation), circulating them, and dissolving the one over the other until they assimilate completely. Afterward, the practitioner must exalt and purify this liquor with spirit of wine and *ennoble, dignify,* and *subtilize* it with spirit of rainwater. Obviously, the metallic principle in this commixture will exist in a much smaller quantity than the menstrual principle. As for the selection of salts and metals, it is unnecessary to go into great detail, since the choice is actually of small importance. However, above all others, we would recommend using the *metallus primus* dissolved in a menstruum of niter prepared with a small portion of common salt.

The practitioner who wishes to prepare an alkahest should first consult Table 17.1 on page 187 to determine which metals can be dissolved by the saline menstrua and metallic mercuries required in the manufacture of alkahests. These salts and metals, when united and exalted spagyrically, are infinitely more powerful than their first natures.

Philosophical Menstrua

We have stated that the elements required in the manufacture of alkahests should be purified and subtilized by spirit of wine, but first it is necessary to obtain the quintessence of this spirit, and to this end we offer, in addition to the spagyric preparations already described, a procedure by which Paracelsus claimed to be able to obtain the spirit of philosophical wine:

Take a certain quantity of very old wine and pour it into a glass vessel, filling only one-third of the vessel. Hermetically seal the receptacle and keep it in horse dung for four months at a continuous heat. Afterward, expose it to the elements for one month during the winter, when the frost and cold are excessive, so that it freezes. Some liquor will remain unfrozen in the center, which is superior to the spirit of wine drawn by fire.[9]

Distillation of Rainwater

Rainwater should be collected at the time of the spring equinox, sometime around May 5, or during the summer. To this end, prepare an open barrel with a handful of salt niter at the bottom and place it in a garden. Wait until the barrel is one-half or three-quarters full and, without worrying whether the water is polluted, keep it exposed to the air for fifteen days. Afterward, filter the water and preserve it in well-sealed bottles of sandstone. This water is better than any other vehicle for the distillation of certain plants and seeds as well as for washing both plants and salts.

To draw from rainwater its volatile spirit, which serves as an admirable menstruum, distill it in a glass or earthenware vessel with a Moor's head and with the serpentine channel passing through the barrel. First, draw only two-thirds, then repeat the distillation until the water reduces to one-tenth of its volume. To obtain the quintessence of this spirit, mix it with an equal portion of putrefied rainwater, distill the spirit again, having poured it back over its water, then, finally, distill the spirit three times by itself to reduce and rectify it. It is with the help of this quintessence that the practitioner may dignify alkahests by repeated circulation and distillation.

Menstrual Acid of Vinegar

Dissolve 1 pound of vinegar crystals or purified tartar in 5 pounds of distilled vinegar and digest them together in a circulatory vessel for two weeks in the steam bath. Next, distill with the retort in the sand bath until desiccated, increasing the fire toward the end of the distillation. Calcine the residue until it turns white, then add another ½ pound of pure tartar. Put these calcined salts in a retort and distill them several times by cohobation, until the spirit raises a large portion of the fixed salt along with it, which will likely happen during the tenth distillation. Lastly, mix this spirit with the first spirit obtained and distill slowly three times, increasing the fire during the final rectification. This menstruum is capable of penetrating metals.

Starkey's Sulfurous Menstruum

Take equal parts dissolved salt of tartar and colcothar of Roman vitriol,* perfectly washed of its salt, and boil them together until the moisture evaporates completely. Melt the mass in the crucible, then pour it out and dissolve it by washing. Next, volatilize this sulfur by mortification and regeneration, then distill and rectify and it will render a yellowish-green balsamic liquor. This liquor can be fixed in the fire with a little prepared mercury, and from this the practitioner may extract an admirable tincture with essential spirit of wine. This tincture is comparable to Helmont's "horizontal gold," which is made by the alkahest.[10]

Philosophical Menstruum for Extracting the Quintessence from Plants

Digest for eight days several kinds of aromatic seeds like anise, cumin, fennel, dill, caraway, nutmeg, mint, and star anise and several kinds of herbs like lemon balm, greater celandine, and mountain arnica with a little salt niter in essential spirit of wine so that the spirit supernates the plant matter. This should be done in the steam bath. Draw the spirit and distill only once. Pour over the plant matter as much volatile spirit of rainwater as there was spirit of wine and digest for four full days in the steam bath. Distill this spirit by cohobating it on the residue three times. Next, mix the two spirits obtained and circulate them in the vessel of Hermes for three days, then distill and rectify one last time.

---

*[The term *colcothar*, which derives from the Greek χάλκανθον, a portmanteau of the words χαλκός, meaning "copper," and ἄνθος, meaning "flower," refers to a copper oxide that is left as a residue when copper sulfate, i.e., *vitriolum Romanum* or "Roman vitriol" (otherwise known as "blue vitriol"), is heated at high temperatures. —*Trans.*]

This plant menstruum is capable of extracting the quintessence from any plant.* Its preparation will not be found in any other work.

Alkahests in Practice

To separate the different principles of a given plant, first wash it with filtered rainwater, then cut it into pieces and put them in a tall and narrow matrass. These pieces should be very dry on the exterior, because the surface water does not form part of the plant's own moisture. Gently pour the alkahest into the matrass so that it rises just above the body of the plant. Seal the matrass and expose it to the light of the Sun or set it in a warm place, in which case the fire of quicklime and hay will suffice. Allow the alkahest to act on the plant matter until various liquors become superimposed in the matrass. The alkahest will show at the bottom in a luminous deep yellow, above it the organic and earthy part of the mixed body in the form of a dark mass, above this a greenish and diaphanous water, and, finally, at the very top, the colored oil, which is the sulfur or essence of the plant. The separation of these principles requires a deft hand.

To divide the principles of a metal, first melt it with niter, bismuth, and borax so that it becomes pure and malleable. When it becomes molten, filter it with a sieve over some cold water to form it into granulated shot. Wash it afterward with boiling water, then dry it and put it in a thick glass matrass. Pour in the alkahest, stop the matrass, and set it to digest in the ash bath until the principles of the metal stratify in various colored liquors, with the earth remaining at the bottom.†

N.B.: For hard parts of plants such as woods, barks, and hard seeds, use simply filtered rainwater or even fountain water in which you have dissolved a little common salt niter. A digestion in one of these vehicles in the steam bath will prepare these hard materials for distillation. Rainwater mixed with cream of tartar will correct mucilaginous purgatives such as senna and rhubarb. The water drawn from the distillation of May dew serves an excellent menstruum that is capable of dissolving gold. Lastly, the *volatile alkali circulated with spirit of wine* is an especially powerful solvent.

†Some claim that the fluorine (F) of modern chemistry was the alkahest of the ancients; see, e.g., Henri Moissan and James Dewar, "On the Properties of Liquid Fluorine," *Proceedings of the Chemical Society* 13 (1897): 175–84. Fluorine is synonymous with phthor, phthore, and phthorine, early names derived from the Greek verb φθείρειν, "to destroy," and all data show that fluorine *destroys* everything it touches. No further comment should be necessary.

Secret Formula for a "Universal *Circulatum*"

Expose to the cool air during the night equal parts of purified salt niter and purified common salt, so that they resolve by deliquium. Desiccate them in the Sun and expose them once more to the cool air of night. Repeat this procedure until they no longer resolve by themselves. Put the salts in a long-necked matrass with a quarter part of tin shavings and pour six parts of ammoniac spirit or "volatile alkali" over the mixture. Expose the well-sealed matrass to a gentle and humid heat for three days. After three days, slowly pour over the alkali some distilled spirit of vinegar until the effervescence ceases. Put all of the contents in a closed vessel and circulate them for seven full days with a slow heat. At the end of seven days, clarify the liquor by filtration and return it to the circulatory with a half part of essential spirit of wine for another seven days.

Next, slowly distill this liquor three times, then mix it with an equal portion of very subtle spirit of rainwater. Let everything circulate for three, seven, or fifteen days, then rectify the solution three times. The quintessential spirit obtained in this manner serves as an admirable noncorrosive solvent that is capable of breaking most mixed bodies down to their primitive elements.

TABLE 17.1.
METALLIC ELEMENTS AND THEIR SOLVENTS

Solvent	Metallic Elements
Menstrual Spirit of Niter	dissolves all metals except tin and gold
Menstrual Spirit of Tartar	dissolves all metals except lead, tin, and antimony
Menstrual Spirit of Common Salt	dissolves iron, tin, and arsenic
Metallus primus	dissolves all metals except iron and bismuth
Glass of Antimony	dissolves all metals except gold
Mercury of Tin	dissolves all metals
Mercury or Quicksilver	dissolves all metals except iron
Mercury of Lead	dissolves all metals except tin, copper, mercury, and silver
Common Sulfur	dissolves all metals except gold and zinc

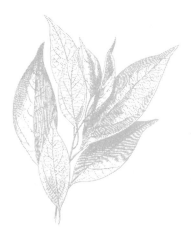

Afterword

Whatever our own knowledge has brought to the production of this work, and despite our concern for its clarity, practitioners will profit from it only insofar as they are capable of penetrating the intimate spirit, for although we have covered every facet of the science of Hermetic herbalism, we have given short shrift to some of the physical aspects of spagyrics. But practical knowledge will flow naturally from theoretical knowledge, which can be assimilated only by those whose faculties are psychically evolved. For this reason, we have directed our efforts primarily toward the study of the intimate, profound, and synthetic nature of the universal laws and their analogies. This, however, is but one part of the art, but it is one which, given its importance and obscurity, practitioners must study in great depth.

Notes

TRANSLATOR'S FOREWORD

1. Mavéric, *L'art métallique des anciens ou l'or artificiel.*
2. Caillet, *Manuel bibliographique des sciences psychiques ou occultes,* 3:60 and 268.
3. Petit, *La clef de l'horoscope quotidien permettant à chacun de suivre jour par jour le cours des astres en prévision des evénéments futurs.*
4. Bélus, *Pour conjurer les sorts et se débarrasser de tous les maux,* and *Traité des recherches.*
5. Diodorus Siculus, *Bibliotheca historica,* 1.28.1 [ed. Vogel-Fischer].
6. Dorbon-aîné, *Bibliotheca esoterica,* 317 no. 3001.
7. See Le Trois Initiés [= W. W. Atkinson], *Le Kybalion.* "Three Initiates" was one of the pseudonyms of William Walker Atkinson (1862–1932).
8. The serial "La médecine spagyrique" appeared in Jollivet-Castelot's journal *Rose + Croix: Revue synthétique des sciences d'Hermès.*
9. Petitjean, *De la hernie inguinale étranglée chez l'enfant dans les deux premières années de sa vie.* See further "Thèses et brochures," *Archives de médecine des enfants* 3 (1900): 313–14; and "Livres," *Journal général de l'imprimerie et de la librairie* 89 no. 13 (1900): 9, no. 3572.
10. Mavéric, *Essai synthétique sur la médecine astrologique et spagyrique.*
11. Duz, *Traité pratique de médecine astrale et de thérapeutique;* translated into English as *A Practical Treatise of Astral Medicine and Therapeutics.*
12. Jollivet-Castelot, review of Jean Mavéric, *La médecine hermétique des plantes,* in *La Rose + Croix: Revue synthétique des sciences d'Hermès* 17 no. 2 (1912): 61–62.

13. The esoteric *chroniqueur* Jacques Brieu expresses the very same sentiments in his review of *Hermetic Herbalism* in "Ésotérisme et sciences psychiques," *Mercure de France* 95, no. 352 (1912): 838–43.

14. Sédir, *Les plantes magiques.* A revised and expanded English translation of this work is in preparation.

AUTHOR'S PREFACE

1. One may note, for example, the published opinions of Georg Ernst Stahl (1659–1734), Paul-Joseph Barthez (1734–1806), François-Joseph-Victor Broussais (1772–1838), Christopher Girtanner (1760–1800), Théophile de Bordeu (1722–1776), François Louis Isidore Valleix (1807–1855), Jean-Emmanuel Gilibert (1741–1814), Johann Peter Frank (1745–1821), François Magendie (1783–1855), Joseph-Claude-Anthelme Récamier (1774–1852), Jacques Etienne Bérard (1789–1869), Philippe Antoine Francoise Barbier (1848–1922), Joseph-François Malgaigne (1806–1865), and Apollinaire Bouchardat (1809–1886), all of which are conveniently summarized in Ponzio's *Traité complet de médecine électro-homéopathique,* 120–26.

INTRODUCTION

1. Vossius, *De vitiis sermonis et glossematis latino-barbaris libri quatuor,* 606: "*Spagirus* Theophrasto Paracelso, pro *alchymista:* unde ars *spagiria,* vel *spagirica.* Puto autem, *spagiricos* dici a duobus artis officiis: quae sunt, composita resolvere, et resoluta componere. Nam σπᾶν, *trahere, extrahere:* ἀγείρειν, *congregare.*"

2. Locques, *Les rudiments de la philosophie naturelle touchant le système du corps mixte,* 199: "*Spargyrie* [*sic*] vient du mot σπάω et ἄγυρος qui enseigne à extraire l'Argent vif des Metaux."

CHAPTER I.
SYNTHESIS OF THE ORIGINS OF CREATION

1. Ettmüller, *Chimia rationalis ac experimentalis curiosa,* 138–40; cf. the French translation published under the title *Nouvelle chymie raisonnée de Michel Ettmüller,* 385–90.

2. Ettmüller, *Chimia rationalis,* 140–41; *Nouvelle chymie raisonnée,* 391–92.

3. Ettmüller, *Chimia rationalis,* 142; *Nouvelle chymie raisonnée,* 394–96.

4. Le Fèvre, *Traicté de la chymie,* 1:260–61; cf. the English translation published under the title *A Compendious Body of Chymistry,* 1:164–65.

5. Le Fèvre, *Traicté de la chymie,* 1:258–61; *A Compendious Body of Chymistry,* 1:163–65.

6. Le Fèvre, *Traicté de la chymie,* 1:261–63; *A Compendious Body of Chymistry,* 1:165–66.

CHAPTER 3. BOERHAAVE'S
CLASSIFICATIONS OF MEDICINAL PLANTS

1. See especially Boerhaave, *Libellus de materie medica et remediorum formulis,* with English translations of various parts and in various editions under the titles *De viribus medicamentorum* (1720), *A Treatise on the Powers of Medicines* (1740), *Materia Medica* (1755), and *Aphorisms concerning the Knowledge and Cure of Diseases* (1755). See also Boerhaave, *Elementa chemiae quae anniversario labore docuit,* and Peter Shaw's English translation under the title *A New Method of Chemistry Including the History, Theory, and Practice of the Art.*

CHAPTER 4.
METHODS OF PLANT PRESERVATION

1. This was the method of Antoine Vallot, first physician to King Louis XIV from 1652 to 1671; cf. Le Fèvre, *Traicté de la chymie,* 1:280; *A Compendious Body of Chymistry,* 1:176–77.

CHAPTER 5.
THE YEAR-ROUND HARVEST

1. Le Fèvre, *Traicté de la chymie,* 1:260; *A Compendious Body of Chymistry,* 1:164.

2. Baumé offers a cogent overview of this subject entitled "Choix de racines" in his *Éléments de pharmacie théorique et pratique,* 1:58–62. Giambattista della Porta says that, in general, roots should be harvested in autumn, flowers in spring, and leaves in summer, and always when the sky is clear

and the weather is calm; see *Magiae naturalis sive de miraculis rerum,*
58–59 (lib. I, cap. XVI: *Simplicia omnia statis exercerci temporibus, et
pariter parari debent*) [English edition: Porta, *Natural Magick,* 20–21
(bk. I, ch. XV: "That all Simples are to be gotten and used in their certain
seasons")].

CHAPTER 6. PLANT SIGNATURES: CORRESPONDENCES OF PLANTS TO THE PLANETS AND THE SIGNS OF THE ZODIAC

1. See further, Mavéric, *Essai synthétique,* 40–41.
2. *Translator's note:* For a concise description of the Doctrine of Signatures as
   it relates to the plant kingdom, see Sédir, *Les plantes magiques,* 39–55. For
   a more detailed analysis of this "Science of Correspondences," see Jollivet-
   Castelot, *La médecine spagyrique.*
3. See Dariot, *De la connaissance des maladies et des jours critiques d'apres le
   mouvement des astres;* cf. Paracelsus, *Der grossen Wundartzney* (French
   edition: *La grand chirurgie de Philippe Aoreole Theophraste Paracelse grand
   médecin et philosophe entre les Alemans*).

CHAPTER 8. PHYSIOLOGICAL AND PSYCHOLOGICAL ANALOGIES OF THE FOUR TEMPERAMENTS

1. *Translator's note:* Mavéric provisionally titled this work *Les grands arcanes
   de la médecine minérale* or "The Great Arcana of Mineral Medicine." At
   the end of the original French publication he announces this work as
   "en préparation," but if he ever completed it, he never published it; see
   *La médecine hermétique des plantes ou l'extraction des quintessences par art
   spagyrique,* 211. Some of Mavéric's ideas on this subject may be gleaned
   from his *L'art métallique des anciens.*

CHAPTER 9. THE HERMETIC DIET

1. Cf. Mavéric, *Essai synthétique,* 96–97.
2. Hermes Trismegistus, *Tabula smaragdina,* line 2 [ed. Ruska].

CHAPTER 10. PLANETARY NATURES
AND THEIR ANALOGIES ON THE
PHYSICAL AND MENTAL PLANES

1. We have no intention here of dealing with the theoretical aspects of astrology. Readers may find all that pertains to the theory and practice of this art in the excellent works of Jules Eveno (alias Julevno), Abel Thomas (alias Abel Haatan), Paul Choisnard (alias Paul Flambart), Charles Nicoullaud (alias Fomalhaut), and Jean (or Joanny) Bricaud. For all that concerns the investigation of diseases in the natal chart, see our *Essai synthétique*, 76–79. Here we focus on all that concerns the Hermetic and medicinal aspects of astrology and discuss only certain discoveries we have made since the conception of our earlier publication.

2. Cf. Mavéric, *Essai synthétique*, 59–60.

3. *Translator's note:* See further Mavéric, *La reforme des bases de l'astrologie traditionelle.*

CHAPTER 11.
MECHANICAL THEORY OF ASTRAL VIBRATIONS

1. Cf. Mavéric, *Essai synthétique*, 82–85.

CHAPTER 12. PRINCIPLES OF PREMODERN CHEMISTRY
FOR BASIC PREPARATIONS OF MEDICINAL PLANTS

1. Glauber, *Furni novi philosophici,* translated into English under the title *A Description of New Philosophical Furnaces;* Nicolas Lémery, *Cours de chymie,* 2nd rev. ed. (1676), translated into English by Walter Harris under the title *A Course of Chymistry* (1677); and Baumé, *Éléments de pharmacie théorique et pratique.*

2. Glaser, *Traité de la chymie,* 324–25; cf. the English translation published under the title *The Compleat Chymist,* 236–37.

3. Glaser, *Traité de la chymie,* 327–30; *The Compleat Chymist,* 238–40.

4. Glaser, *Traité de la chymie,* 330–32; *The Compleat Chymist,* 240–41.

5. Glaser, *Traité de la chymie,* 332–34; *The Compleat Chymist,* 241–42.

6. Glaser, *Traité de la chymie,* 335–38; *The Compleat Chymist,* 243–45.

7. Glaser, *Traité de la chymie,* 338–41; *The Compleat Chymist,* 245–46.

CHAPTER 13. PLANT JUICES AND THEIR USES

1. Glaser, *Traité de la chymie*, 369–70; *The Compleat Chymist*, 267–68.
2. Glaser, *Traité de la chymie*, 371–72; *The Compleat Chymist*, 268–69.
3. Cox, "A Way of Extracting a Volatile Salt and Spirit out of Vegetables," 4–8.
4. Glaser, *Traité de la chymie*, 298–301; *The Compleat Chymist*, 219–21.
5. Glaser, *Traité de la chymie*, 366–68; *The Compleat Chymist*, 265–66.
6. Glaser, *Traité de la chymie*, 289–92; *The Compleat Chymist*, 213–14.
7. Glaser, *Traité de la chymie*, 292–93; *The Compleat Chymist*, 215.
8. Glaser, *Traité de la chymie*, 293–95; *The Compleat Chymist*, 216–17.
9. Glaser, *Traité de la chymie*, 301–4; *The Compleat Chymist*, 221–23.
10. Glaser, *Traité de la chymie*, 306–7; *The Compleat Chymist*, 224–25.
11. Glaser, *Traité de la chymie*, 311–12; *The Compleat Chymist*, 227–28.
12. Glaser, *Traité de la chymie*, 315–17; *The Compleat Chymist*, 230–31.
13. Glaser, *Traité de la chymie*, 320–23; *The Compleat Chymist*, 233–35.
14. See Quesnot, *Plusieurs secrets rares et curieux pour la guérison des maladies*, 198–209; cf. Le Fèvre, *Cours de la chimie pour servir d'introduction à cette science*, 410–11.

CHAPTER 14.
LE FÈVRE'S CHEMICAL PREPARATIONS OF PLANTS

1. Le Fèvre, *Traicté de la chymie*, 1:264–72; *A Compendious Body of Chymistry*, 1:167–71.
2. Le Fèvre, *Traicté de la chymie*, 1:272–74; *A Compendious Body of Chymistry*, 1:171–73.
3. Le Fèvre, *Traicté de la chymie*, 1:274–82; *A Compendious Body of Chymistry*, 1:173–77.
4. Le Fèvre, *Traité de la chymie*, 211–12.
5. Le Fèvre, *Traité de la chymie*, 213–14.
6. Le Fèvre, *Traicté de la chymie*, 1:375–81; *A Compendious Body of Chymistry*, 1:232–36.
7. Le Fèvre, *Traicté de la chymie*, 1:381–82; *A Compendious Body of Chymistry*, 1:236–38.
8. Le Fèvre, *Traicté de la chymie*, 1:383–86; *A Compendious Body of Chymistry*, 1:238–39.

9. Le Fèvre, *Traicté de la chymie,* 1:386–88; *A Compendious Body of Chymistry,* 1:239–40.

10. Le Fèvre, *Traicté de la chymie,* 1:442–47; *A Compendious Body of Chymistry,* 1:271–74.

11. Le Fèvre, *Traicté de la chymie,* 1:492–93; *A Compendious Body of Chymistry,* 1:301–2.

12. Le Fèvre, *Traicté de la chymie,* 1:282–84; *A Compendious Body of Chymistry,* 1:177–79.

13. Le Fèvre, *Traicté de la chymie,* 1:284–85; *A Compendious Body of Chymistry,* 1:179.

14. Le Fèvre, *Traicté de la chymie,* 1:290–91; *A Compendious Body of Chymistry,* 1:182.

15. Le Fèvre, *Traicté de la chymie,* 1:291; *A Compendious Body of Chymistry,* 1:183.

CHAPTER 15.
INTRODUCTION TO THE SPAGYRIC ART

1. Barlet, *Le vray et methodique cours de la physique resolutive, vulgairement dite chymie,* 162.

2. Cf. Paracelsus, *The Hermetic and Alchemical Writings of Paracelsus the Great,* 2:33–34.

3. Reutter de Rosemont, *Histoire de la pharmacie à travers les âges,* 1:593.

4. Ulstad, *Coelum philosophorum,* 152–61 (cap. XVI); cf. *Le ciel des philosophes, où sont contenus les secretz de nature, et comme l'homme se peult tenir en santé, et longuement vivre,* 91r–92v (ch. 16).

5. Le Fèvre, *Traicté de la chymie,* 1:282–84; *A Compendious Body of Chymistry,* 1:177–79.

6. Rosemont, *Histoire de la pharmacie à travers les âges,* 1:593.

7. Pseudo-Llull, "Aqua duplicativa," 210.

8. Cf. Pseudo-Llull, *De secretis natvrae, sev de quinta essentia liber vnus, in tres distinctiones diuisus, omnibus iam partibus absolutus,* 26.

9. Pseudo-Llull, "Ars operativa medica," 182.

10. Ulstad, *Coelum philosophorum,* 327–28 (cap. XLV); *Le ciel des philosophes,* 81v–82r (ch. 45).

11. Ulstad, *Coelum philosophorum,* 328–31 (cap. XLVI); *Le ciel des philosophes,* 82r–83r (ch. 46).

12. Ulstad, *Coelum philosophorum*, 360–62 (cap. LVII); *Le ciel des philosophes*, 91r–92v (ch. 57).

13. Croll, *Basilica chymica*, 146–47; cf. the English translation published under the title *Bazilica chymica*, 49–50.

14. Gessner, *Thesaurus Euonymi Philiatri de remediis secretis*, 148–52; cf. the French and English translations published under the titles *Tresor des remedes secretz*, 130–32, and *The Treasure of Euonymus conteyninge the Vvonderfull Hid Secretes of Nature*, 107–8.

15. Pseudo-Llull, *De secretis naturae*, 118–19.

16. Le Fèvre, *Traicté de la chimie*, 2:757–60; *A Compendious Body of Chymistry*, 2:110–12.

17. Brosse, *A Monseigneur le tres-illustre et le tres-reverend Cardinal, Monseigneur le Cardinal de Richelieu, à propos du jardin des plantes*, 9–10.

CHAPTER 16. THE SPAGYRIC MEDICINES OF PARACELSUS AND HELMONT

1. Helmont, "Vita aeterna," in *Ortus medicinae*, 741–43.

2. Starkey, *Nature's Explication and Helmont's Vindication*, 313–19.

3. Starkey, *Pyrotechny Asserted and Illustrated*, 127–28.

CHAPTER 17. THE ART OF VOLATILIZING ALKALIS

1. See Starkey, *Pyrotechny Asserted and Illustrated*, 151–56.

2. *Translator's note*: This quotation is Mavéric's adaptation of passages from Jean Le Pelletier's freely revised and abridged translation of Starkey's *Pyrotechny*, 28, 120; see *La pyrotecnie de Starkey*, 71–72.

3. Le Pelletier, *L'alkaest*.

4. Paracelsus, *De viribus membrorum*, lib. II, cap. VI (*De cura hepatis*). For an English translation of this work, see *Paracelsus, His Archidoxis*, 61–90.

5. See Dorn, *Dictionarium Theophrasti Paracelsi*, 14 s.v. *Alcahest*; and Ruland, *Lexicon alchemiae siue dictionarium alchemisticum*, 26 s.v. *Alcahest*.

6. Paracelsus, *The Hermetic and Alchemical Writings of Paracelsus*, 2:86.

7. Cf. Paracelsus, *The Hermetic and Alchemical Writings*, 2:15.

8. Cf. Paracelsus, *The Hermetic and Alchemical Writings*, 2:30–31.

9. Cf. Paracelsus, *The Hermetic and Alchemical Writings*, 2:56–57.

10. Starkey, *Pyrotechny*, 83–84.

Bibliography

Atkinson, William Walker. *Le Kybalion: Étude sur la philosophie hermétique de l'ancienne Egypte et de l'ancienne Grèce.* Translated by André Durville with a preface by Albert Louis Caillet. Paris: Durville, 1917.

Barlet, Annibal. *Le vray et méthodique cours de la physique résolutive, vulgairement dite chymie.* Paris: Charles, 1653.

Baumé, Antoine. *Éléments de pharmacie théorique et pratique.* 8th ed. 2 vols. Paris: Magasin de Librairie, 1797.

Bélus, Jean. *Pour conjurer les sorts et se débarrasser de tous les maux. Paris: Société française, 1911.*

———. *Traité des recherches, pour la découverte des personnes disparues, des enfants, animaux et objets perdus ou volés.* Paris: Ficker, 1911.

Berthelot, Marcellin. *Les origines de l'alchimie.* Paris: Steinheil, 1885.

Boerhaave, Herman. *A New Method of Chemistry Including the History, Theory, and Practice of the Art.* 3rd ed. Translated by Peter Shaw. London: Osborn and Longman, 1753.

———. *Aphorisms concerning the Knowledge and Cure of Diseases.* London: Innys, 1755.

———. *A Treatise on the Powers of Medicines.* London: Wilcox, 1740.

———. *Elementa chemiae quae anniversario labore docuit, in publicis, privatisque scholis, Hermannus Boerhaave.* 2 vols. Leiden: Severinus, 1732.

———. *Libellus de materie medica et remediorum formulis, quae serviunt aphorismis de cognoscendis et curandis morbis.* Leiden: Severinus, 1727.

———. *De viribus medicamentorum or a Treatise of the Virtue and Energy of Medicines.* London: Wilcox, 1720.

———. *Materia Medica or the Druggist's Guide and the Physician and the Apothecary's Table-Book*. London: Hodges, 1755.

Brieu, Jacques. "Ésotérisme et sciences psychiques." *Mercure de France* 95, no. 352 (1912): 838–43.

Brosse, Guy de la. *A Monseigneur le très-illustre et le très-révérend Cardinal, Monseigneur le Cardinal de Richelieu, à propos du jardin des plantes*. s.l.: s.n., 1620.

Caillet, Albert Louis. *Manuel bibliographique des sciences psychiques ou occultes*. 3 vols. Paris: Dorbon, 1912.

Chambaud, Louis. *The Idioms of the French and English Languages*. London: Symonds, 1793.

Cox, Daniel. "A Way of Extracting a Volatile Salt and Spirit out of Vegetables." *Philosophical Transactions* 9 (1674): 4–8.

Croll, Oswald. *Basilica chymica: Continens philosophicam propria laborum experientia confirmatam descriptionem et usum remediorum chymicorum*. Frankfurt am Main: Marinus and Aubrius, 1609.

———. *Bazilica chymica et Praxis chymiatricae, or Royal and Practical Chymistry in Three Treatises*. London: Starkey, 1670.

Culpeper, Nicholas. *The Complete Herbal: To Which is Now Added, Upwards of One Hundred Additional Herbs, with a Display of their Medicinal and Occult Qualities, Physically Applied to the Cure of All Disorders Incident to Mankind*. London: Kelly, 1843.

Dariot, Claude. *De la connaissance des maladies et des jours critiques d'apres le mouvement des astres*. Lyon: s.n., 1582.

Dorbon-aîné. *Bibliotheca esoterica: Catalogue annoté et illustré de 6707 ouvrages anciens et modernes, qui traitent des sciences occultes (alchimie, astrologie, cartomancie, chiromancie, démonologie, grimoires, hypnotisme, kabbale, magie, magnétisme, médicine spagirique, mysticisme, prophéties, recettes et secrets, sorcellerie, spiritisme, théosophie, etc.), comme aussi de sociétés secrétes (franc-maçonnerie, rose-croix, templiers, compagnonnage, illuminés, hérésies, etc.)*. Paris: Dorbon-aîné, 1940.

Dorn, Gerhard. *Dictionarium Theophrasti Paracelsi, continens obscuriorum vocabulorum, quibus in suis scriptis passim vtitur, definitiones*. Frankfurt am Main: Rab, 1583.

Duz, M. *Traité pratique de médecine astrale et de thérapeutique*. Paris: La médicine pratique, 1910.

———. *A Practical Treatise of Astral Medicine and Therapeutics*. London: Foulsham, 1912.

Ettmüller, Michael. *Chimia rationalis ac experimentalis curiosa.* Leiden: s.n., 1684.

———. *Nouvelle chymie raisonnée de Michel Ettmüller, célèbre médecin et professeur de l'Université de Leipsik.* Lyon: Amaulry, 1693.

Gessner, Conrad. *Thesaurus Euonymi Philiatri de remediis secretis.* Lyon: Arnoulletus, 1554.

———. *The Treasure of Euonymus conteyninge the Vvonderfull Hid Secretes of Nature.* Translated by Peter Morvvying. London: Daie, 1559.

———. *Tresor des remedes secretz: Livre physic, medical, alchymic, et dispensatif de toutes substantiales liqueurs, et appareil de vins de diverses saveurs.* Translated by Barthélemy Aneau. Lyon: Arnoullet, 1557.

Glaser, Christophe. *Traité de la chymie: Enseignant par une briéve et facile methode toutes ses plus necessaire preparations.* 3rd rev. ed. Lyon: Thioly, 1670.

———. *The Compleat Chymist, or A New Treatise of Chymistry, Teaching by a Short and Easy Method All Its Most Necessary Preparations.* Translated by "a Fellow of the Royal Society." London: Starkey, 1677.

Glauber, Rudolf. *A Description of New Philosophical Furnaces, or A New Art of Distilling.* London: Coats, 1651.

———. *Furni novi philosophici, sive descriptio artis destillatoriae novae.* Amsterdam: Jansson, 1651.

Helmont, Jan Baptist van. *Ortus medicinae, id est, Initia physicæ inaudita: Progressus medicinae novus, in morborum ultionem ad vitam longam.* Amsterdam: Elzevirius, 1648.

Jollivet-Castelot, François. *La médecine spagyrique: Oswald Crollius, Joseph du Chesne, Jean d'Aubry, avec la réédition intégrale du traité des signatures et correspondances de Crollius.* Paris: Durville, 1912.

———. Review of Jean Mavéric, *La médecine hermétique des plantes. La Rose + Croix: Revue synthétique des sciences d'Hermès* 17, no. 2 (1912): 61–62.

Le Fèvre, Nicaise. *A Compendious Body of Chymistry, Teaching the Whole Practice Thereof by the Most Exact Preparation of Animals, Vegetables and Minerals, Preserving their Essential Virtues.* 2 vols. London: Davies and Sadler, 1662.

———. *Cours de la chimie pour servir d'introduction à cette science.* Paris: Leloup, 1751.

———. *Traicté de la chymie.* 2 vols. Paris: Jolly, 1660.

———. *Traité de la chymie.* 2 vols. 2nd rev. ed. Paris: d'Houry, 1674.

Lémery, Nicolas. *A Course of Chymistry: Containing an Easie Method of*

Preparing Those Chymical Medicines Which are Used in Physick. Translated by Walter Harris. London: Bell, 1677.

———. *Cours de chymie: Contenant la manière de faire les opérations qui sont en usage dans la médecine, par une méthode facile.* 2nd rev. ed. Paris: Lémery, 1676.

Le Pelletier, Jean. *L'alkaest, ou le dissolvant universal de Van-Helmont: Revelé dans plusieurs traitez qui en découvrent le secret.* Rouen: Behourt, 1706.

Libavius, Andreas. *De theriaca Andromachi senioris, ex Mithridatio nata, et a temporibus Neronis Principis in Imperio Romano per Graecos et Lationos Medicos celebrata.* Coburg: Bertsch, 1613.

Lindsay, W. M., ed. *Isidori Hispalensis episcopi Etymologiarum sive Originvm libri XX.* Oxford: Clarendon, 1911.

Locques, Nicolas de. *Les rudiments de la philosophie naturelle touchant le système du corps mixte.* Paris: Marcher, 1665.

Mavéric, Jean. *Essai synthétique sur la médecine astrologique et spagyrique.* Paris: Vigot frères, 1910.

———. *La médecine hermétique des plantes ou l'extraction des quintessences par art spagyrique.* Paris: Dorbon-aîné, 1911.

———. *La reforme des bases de l'astrologie traditionelle.* Paris: Leclerc, 1912.

———. *L'art métallique des anciens ou l'or artificiel: Génération de l'or et des métaux ou les opérations les plus curieuses de l'art.* Paris: Siéver, 1910.

Moissan, Henri, and James Dewar. "On the Properties of Liquid Fluorine." *Proceedings of the Chemical Society* 13 (1897): 175–84.

Paracelsus (Theophrast von Hohenheim). *Paracelsus, His Archidoxis, Comprised in Ten Books, Disclosing the Genuine Way of Making Quintessences, Arcanums, Magisteries, Elixirs, etc., Together with His Books, Of Renovation and Restauration, Of the Tincture of the Philosophers, Of the Manual of the Philosophical Medicinal Stone, Of the Virtues of the Members, Of the Three Principles, and Finally His Seven Books, Of the Degrees and Compositions of Receipts and Natural Things.* London: Brewster, 1660.

———. *La grand chirurgie de Philippe Aoreole Theophraste Paracelse grand médecin et philosophe entre les Alemans.* Translated by Claude Dariot. Lyon: de Harsy, 1589.

———. *Der grossen Wundartzney.* Augspurg: Steyner, 1536.

———. *The Hermetic and Alchemical Writings of Paracelsus the Great.* 2 vols. Translated by Arthur Edward Waite. London: Elliott, 1894.

Petit, Jean. *La clef de l'horoscope quotidien permettant à chacun de suivre jour par jour le cours des astres en prévision des evénéments futurs.* Paris: Durville, 1913.

Petitjean, Maurice. *De la hernie inguinale étranglée chez l'enfant dans les deux premières années de sa vie.* Paris: Vigot frères, 1899.

Ponzio, Pierre Louis. *Traité complet de médecine électro-homéopathique: Pathologie nouvelle—therapeutique nouvelle.* Paris: Baillière, 1889.

Porta, Giambattista della. *Natural Magick by John Baptista Porta.* London: Young and Speed, 1658.

———. *Magiae naturalis sive de miraculis rerum naturalium libri IV.* Antwerp: Plantin, 1564.

Pseudo-Llull. "Aqua duplicativa." In *Ioannis de Rvpescissa qvi ante CCCXX. annos vixit, de consideratione Quintae essentie rerum omnium, opus sane egregium,* 208–36. Basil: s.n., 1561.

———. "Ars operativa medica." In *Ioannis de Rvpescissa qvi ante CCCXX. annos vixit, de consideratione Quintae essentie rerum omnium, opus sane egregium,* 175–208. Basil: s.n., 1561.

———. *De secretis naturae, seu de quinta essentia liber unus, in tres distinctiones divisus, omnibus iam partibus absolutus.* Cologne: Birckmann, 1567.

Quesnot. *Plusieurs secrets rares et curieux pour la guérison des maladies, pour la metallique, l'oeconomique et les teintures, la medecine du Flos-coeli et autres curiositez.* Paris: Aubouyn, 1708.

Quincy, John. *Pharmacopoeia officinalis & extemporanea, or A Compleat English Dispensatory in Four Parts.* 2nd ed. London: Bell, Taylor, and Osborn, 1719.

Reutter de Rosemont, Louis. *Histoire de la pharmacie à travers les âges.* 2 vols. Paris: Peyronnet, 1931–1932.

Ruland, Martin. *Lexicon alchemiae sive dictionarium alchemisticum: Cum obscuriorum verborum, et rerum hermeticarum, tum Theophrast-Paracelsicarum phrasium, planam explicationem continens.* Frankfurt am Main: Zacharias Palthenius, 1612.

Ruska, Julius, ed. *Tabula smaragdina: Ein Beitrag zur Geschichte der hermetischen Literatur.* Edited by Julius Ruska. Heidelberger Akten der Von-Portheim-Stiftung 16. Heidelberg: Winter, 1926.

Sédir, Paul. *Les plantes magiques: Botanique occulte, constitution sècrete des végétaux vertus des simples, médecine hermétique, philtres, onguents, breuvages magiques, teintures, arcanes, élixirs spagyriques.* Paris: Bibliothèque Chacornac, 1902.

Starkey, George. *Nature's Explication and Helmont's Vindication, or A Short and Sure Way to a Long and Sound Life.* London: Cotes, 1657.

———. *Pyrotechny Asserted and Illustrated: To Be the Surest and Safest Means for the Art's Triumph over Nature's Infirmities.* London: Whitwood, 1696.

———. *La pyrotecnie de Starkey, ou l'art de volatiliser les alcalis, selon les preceptes de Vanhelmont, et la préparation des remedes succedanées ou aprochans de ceux que l'on peut préparer par l'alkaest.* Translated by Jean Le Pelletier. Rouen: Behourt, 1706.

Ulstad, Philipp. *Coelum philosophorum, seu liber de secretis naturae.* Lyons: Rouillius, 1553.

———. *Le ciel des philosophes, où sont contenus les secretz de nature, et comme l'homme se peult tenir en santé, et longuement vivre.* Paris: Gaultherot, 1546.

Vogel, Friedrich, and Curt Theodor Fischer, eds. *Diodori Bibliotheca historica.* Leipzig: Teubner, 1890–1906.

Vossius, Gerardus Johannes. *De vitiis sermonis et glossematis latino-barbaris libri quatuor.* Amsterdam: Elzevirius, 1645.

Index of Common
Plant Names

Index of Scientific
Plant Names

Hedera (ivy), 21, 46
Helleborus foetidus (stinking hellebore),
170
Hepatica (liverwort), 20, 28
Heracleum sphondylium (hogweed), 21
Herniaria glabra (smooth rupturewort),
18
Herniaria hirsuta (hairy rupturewort),
27, 34
Hibiscus (rose mallow), 24, 28
Hieracium (hawkweed), 26
Hieracium pilosella (mouse-ear
hawkweed), 21
Hordeum distichum (barley), 21, 26, 31,
63, 65
Humulus lupulus (common hop), 12,
20, 26, 33, 44
Hydrocotyle vulgaris (marsh
pennywort), 22
Hyoscyamus niger (henbane), 22, 24, 34,
44, 170
Hypericum perforatum (Saint John's
wort), 21, 23, 26–27, 34, 45–46,
125, 152
Hyssopus officinalis (hyssop), 19, 25, 31,
34, 43, 46, 148–49

Ilex (holly), 21
Illicium verum (star anise), 20, 26,
45–46, 185
Inula helenium (elecampane), 17, 23,
35, 124–25, 170, 176
Ipomoea batatas (sweet potato), 24
Ipomoea macrorhiza (largeroot morning
glory)
plant, 113
root (mechoacan), 113
Ipomoea purga (jalap), 43, 101, 112–13,
170, 176
Iris (iris), 17, 25, 27, 33, 43
Iris pseudacorus (yellow iris), 21

Isatis tinctoria (wild woad), 22

Jacobaea vulgaris (common ragwort), 21
Jasminum officinale (jasmine), 13, 30, 44
Juglans (walnut), 18, 33–34, 63–64
Juniperus communis (juniper), 18,
25–28, 32, 35, 37, 46–47, 109,
111–12, 134, 139n, 149, 156
Juniperus sabina (savin), 18, 24, 28, 34,
44, 47

Kali turgidum (prickly saltwort), 21
Knautia (scabious), 18, 24–25, 27–28,
34, 45
Krameria (rhatany), 43

Lactuca (lettuce), 12–13, 22, 24,
26–28, 36–37, 39, 64, 103–4, 112,
152
Lactuca sativa (romaine), 12, 22, 37,
39, 64
Lamium album (white nettle), 33
Lapsana (nipplewort), 21
Laserpitium siler (laserwort), 27
Lathyrus linifolius (bitter vetch), 21, 34
Laurus nobilis (bay laurel), 19, 25, 27,
44, 46
Lavandula (lavender), 13, 19, 25, 30,
34, 47, 148–51
Lavandula dentata (French lavender),
34
Lavandula latifolia (spike lavender), 151
Lemna minor (common duckweed), 22
Lens culinaris (lentil), 22, 31, 63, 65
Leontopodium alpinum (edelweiss), 24,
27, 34
Leonurus cardiaca (motherwort), 19,
24, 28
Lepidium (pepper cress), 20, 24
Lepidium sativum (garden cress),
123–24

Rumex acetosa (sorrel), 12, 18, 23, 26–27, 33, 64, 104–5
Rumex crispus (curly dock), 43
Rumex hydrolapathum (water dock), 20
Rumex sanguineus (bloody dock), 20, 23
Ruscus aculeatus (butcher's broom), 18, 25–26, 33, 35, 147
Ruta graveolens (rue), 18, 24, 27–28, 33, 45–46, 118, 148–51

Salix (willow), 22
Salvia (sage), 13, 19, 25, 27–28, 30, 34, 43, 47, 110, 148–51
Salvia sclarea (clary sage), 34
Sambucus (elderberry), 17, 24, 26, 28, 33, 35, 38, 45
Sambucus ebulus (dwarf elder), 17, 47, 111
Sanguisorba minor (salad burnet), 21, 23, 148, 152
Sanicula europaea (wood sanicle), 21, 28, 34
Santalum (sandalwood), 19, 28, 160
Santolina (santolina), 20
Saponaria officinalis (common soapwort), 21, 23, 34, 44
Sassafras (sassafras), 26
Satureja hortensis (savory), 19, 24–25, 45, 148
Satyrium (satyrion), 19, 24–25, 33, 126, 176
Saxifraga (saxifrage), 33
Scilla (squill), 19, 24–25, 28
Scorzonera hispanica (black salsify), 18, 24, 26, 28
Scrophularia (figwort), 25, 33–34, 44
Scrophularia canina (dog figwort), 21
Scrophularia nodosa (common figwort), 21, 46
Secale cereale (rye), 22, 31, 63, 65, 125–26

Sedum (stonecrop), 21, 24
Sedum album (white stonecrop), 24, 153n
Sedum telephium (orpine), 24
Semecarpus anacardium (bhilawa), 43
Sempervivum (houseleek), 12, 22, 108–9, 153n
Sempervivum tectorum (common houseleek), 23
Seneco vulgaris (groundsel), 21, 34, 36–37
Senegalia catechu (catechu), 20
Senna (senna), 17, 44, 186n
Seseli (hartwort), 20, 34
Seseli tortuosum (Massilian hartwort), 26
Silene coronaria (rose campion), 18
Silybum marianum (milk thistle), 12, 18, 24
Simarouba (simarouba), 17, 26
Sinapis (mustard), 12–13, 17, 24, 26, 63, 109, 122
Sison amomum (stone parsley), 20, 122
Sisymbrium officinale (hedge mustard), 17, 24–25, 122
Sium (water parsnip), 20, 24, 26, 28, 122
Sium sisarum (skirret), 18
Smilax (greenbrier), 26
Smilax ornata (sarsaparilla), 18, 26, 44
Smyrnium olusatrum (Alexanders), 18
Solanum dulcamara (bittersweet), 22, 43
Solanum lycopersicum (tomato), 22–23, 64
Solanum melongena (eggplant), 22, 64
Solanum nigrum (black nightshade), 24–25, 34, 153n
Solanum tuberosum (potato), 35, 63–64
Solidago virgaurea (goldenrod), 21, 27, 46, 125

Index of
Authors and Subjects